Gluten

C000050082

Facts and Truths About: Gluten, Eating Paleo, Celiac Disease, and Related Conditions

5th Edition

By

Arianna Brooks

Arianna Brooks

Table of Contents

Introduction

You may have often heard or read about the gluten-free diet, but not many people may be aware of what gluten is or why people all over the world are avoiding the consumption of food products that contain gluten.

To put it simply, gluten is a type of protein that is found in grains. So, why are a lot of people avoiding this protein? Well, a lot of people (more like 1 in 100 people) are allergic to this particular protein, and it can wreak a considerable amount of havoc in their bodies.

Many people believe that following a gluten-free diet helps make weight loss easier. This may be because most high-calorie foods contain grains or products derived from grains. Thus, when you follow a gluten-free diet, you are forced to avoid these foods and eat healthier. This results in a healthier you!

In the first chapter of this book, I will explain what gluten is, what the main sources of gluten are, and why it is important to avoid gluten. You will also learn about the different symptoms of and emotional responses to gluten intolerance.

The second chapter contains information about what exactly a gluten-free diet is and how you can easily adjust to this restrictive diet.

In the third chapter, I will share what eating Paleo is and how it fits in with a gluten-free way of life. Moreover, I will discuss the nutrition that you can and will receive while following Paleo, the foods that you can consume and those that you should avoid while eating Paleo, as well as the pros and cons of Paleo. You will also find some exercises and workout regimes you can use when you follow the diet. The book also has information about the different steps you can take to ease into the diet.

Additional chapters contain details about what celiac disease is, how it can be diagnosed, its long-term effects on the body, and the ways by which the disease is treated. The book likewise sheds some light on how you should read nutrition fact labels on the products you purchase. You need to do this, especially if you want to lead a healthy life. The book has information on how you can understand these labels and leaves you with some tips you can use to know the ingredients better. It also provides information on gluten intolerance and some of its symptoms. It is important to learn this information, especially if you want to find a way to overcome it.

You will also learn about maintaining a gluten-free lifestyle and the types of food you need to purchase. The book includes a chapter on the different substitutes you need to ensure you stick to a healthy diet. Use these suggestions to help you stick to a healthier eating pattern. It also has information about the different products you should consider when you follow a gluten-free diet. It is difficult for people to follow and maintain a gluten-free diet when they go out or travel. This book provides some tips to help you deal with this.

The final chapters contain a large number of breakfast, lunch, dinner, appetizer, side dish, and dessert recipes that you can use in your day-to-day life. These recipes are easy and quick to make, and all the ingredients required for these recipes can easily be found in most supermarkets, if not in most pantries! There is also a bonus chapter at the end of the book with a sample meal plan you can use to help you ease into the diet.

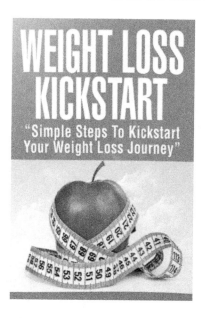

Arianna Brooks

Chapter 1: Gluten – What It Is and Why You Need to Avoid It

What Is Gluten?

Gluten refers to the protein present in most grains, especially in barley, wheat, rye, and triticale. The gluten present in foods helps keep the food together and helps the food maintain its shape. Gluten can be found in many food types.

The 4 Main Sources of Gluten

Wheat

Wheat is one of the most commonly used grains and one of the main sources of gluten in a regular diet. You may not even notice that wheat or wheat-related products are creeping into your diet! Below is a list of some of the products that contain wheat or wheat products, unless specifically mentioned otherwise.

- Cereals
- Fresh or dried pasta
- Breads
- Sauces
- Baked goods
- Salad dressings

- Canned or tinned soups

- Roux

Barley

Barley was one of the first grains cultivated by man. Today, it has become one of the most widely cultivated grains in the world. This means that many prepackaged products and precooked foods may have varying amounts of barley in them, unless otherwise specified. Below is a list of some of these foods.

- Food coloring

- Malt

- Beer

- Malt vinegar

- Soups

Rye

Rye is a cover crop related to both wheat and barley. Although rye is usually grown as fodder, it is also used in a wide variety of breads and alcoholic beverages. Below is a list of items that may contain rye, unless otherwise specified.

- Rye beer

- Crisp bread

- Rye bread

- Certain whiskeys

- Cereals

- Certain vodkas

Triticale

Triticale is a "new" hybrid grain created by combining wheat and rye. This grain was designed to withstand a large variety of growing conditions. Triticale can usually be found in foods like the following:

- Pasta

- Breads

- Cereals

Reasons to Avoid Consuming Foods that Contain Gluten

Gluten is a type of protein that helps food maintain its shape. Pretty harmless, right? So, why is the "gluten-free diet" a rising fad across the world? Here are a few of the reasons why you should avoid anything and everything with gluten in it like the plague!

- Gluten has inflammatory properties that have caused gut inflammation in at least 80% of people. Moreover, the gut develops antibodies against gluten in close to 30% of the population.

- When the gut does not exhibit this reaction against gluten, it is released into the bloodstream where it triggers such reactions somewhere else in the body.

- Gliadin, the gluten protein that causes problems in the body, has a structure that is very similar to that of the tissues in the pancreas and the thyroid. Thus, the antibodies that are built against gliadin in the body end up attacking the thyroid and the pancreas, resulting in autoimmune diseases like diabetes and hypothyroidism.

- The inflammatory properties of gluten in the gut also result in the premature oxidation of cells in the intestine and result in cell death. This causes the weakening of the gut, which may result in the release of bacteria and other toxic components into the bloodstream. This condition further leads to a variety of other autoimmune diseases.

- A weakened gut also results in the partial digestion of food and restricted absorption of nutrients into the body, which may lead to deficiencies related to a number of important nutrients.

- The anti-gluten antibodies produced by the body have also been known to attack the tissues of the heart, thus resulting in a variety of cardiovascular problems.

- Gluten has potential cancer-causing properties, and it promotes cancerous growth in the body.

Apart from all of that, there's another set of problems that arise from gluten, and such problems can be grouped into the category of gluten allergy.

Gluten Allergy

In the past, allergy stemming from gluten and any intolerance toward it were viewed as rare disorders with low incidence. Even now, many people are not aware of these disorders and are often under diagnosed or misdiagnosed as a result.

Causes

- Consuming foods that are ingestible and using antibiotics can damage the intestinal probiotic bacteria.

- Some people even have a gene that can cause their immune system to react to gluten as if it's a microbial invader.

- As a result of diets with low nutritional value, interference in the process of suppressing specific immune cells that attack benign proteins may occur.

- Digesting grains is difficult for infants. There could be an increase of risk in dysbiosis, manifesting if they are fed these grains well before time. The damage to gut flora is called dysbiosis, which is another cause of gluten allergy.

The points mentioned above are just a few possible scenarios as to why someone may develop a gluten allergy or intolerance toward it. However, it isn't necessary for one or more of the points mentioned to be present in someone's life for him or her to suffer from gluten intolerance or allergy.

Symptoms of Gluten Intolerance

Gluten intolerance is a common problem. It is characterized by a terrible reaction to gluten, which is a protein found in barley, rye, and wheat.

Celiac disease is a severe form of gluten intolerance. It is an autoimmune disease that affects at least 1% of the population. It can cause some damage to the digestive system.

Some people are sensitive to gluten but do not have celiac disease, but this still causes some problems. These are common forms of gluten intolerance, but these do not necessarily lead to digestive problems. The following are some common symptoms of gluten intolerance:

Bloating

If your belly feels swollen or full of gas after you eat, it means you are bloated. This will make you feel terrible. Bloating is very common, and there can be various explanations for why this happens. One of the signs can be gluten intolerance. People who are intolerant or sensitive to gluten may often feel bloated, which is a common complaint. A study conducted by Volta U et al. in 2014 showed that at least 87% of people experienced bloating, and they suspected they were intolerant to gluten.

Smelly Feces, Diarrhea, and Constipation

It is normal for people to feel constipated and experience diarrhea, but this becomes a concern if it is a regular occurrence. These are common symptoms of celiac disease and gluten intolerance.

If you have celiac disease, you may experience some inflammation in your small intestine when you eat gluten. This causes damage to your intestine, especially the lining, which reduces its ability to absorb nutrients. This will result in frequent constipation, diarrhea, and digestive discomfort.

Even if you do not have celiac disease, you may have some trouble with digestion when you eat food with gluten. Over 50% of people who are intolerant to gluten regularly experience diarrhea, and 25% experience constipation.

If you have celiac disease, you may experience foul-smelling feces because of poor nutrient absorption. Diarrhea can also cause some health issues, such as dehydration, fatigue, and loss of electrolytes.

Abdominal Pain

There can be various reasons for abdominal pain. This is one of the most common symptoms of gluten intolerance or celiac disease. At least 83% of people with gluten intolerance experience discomfort after eating food with gluten. They may also experience abdominal pain and cramps.

Migraines and Headaches

Most people experience migraines and headaches frequently or occasionally, depending on the amount of stress they are under. Migraines are very common, and at least 12% of the American population experience them regularly. A study conducted by Dimitrova A K et al. in 2013 concluded that people with gluten intolerance and celiac disease are prone to migraines as compared to others. If you experience headaches without any cause, it can be because of gluten sensitivity.

Exhaustion and Tiredness

It is very common for you to feel tired and exhausted, but this is not related to a disease. If you feel tired constantly, you need to understand the underlying cause. If you are intolerant to gluten, you are prone to feeling tired and exhausted, especially after eating food with gluten. A study conducted by Volta U et al. in 2014 showed that people who are intolerant to gluten commonly experience fatigue and tiredness. Gluten intolerance also causes anemia, which leads to a lack of energy and increased tiredness.

Skin Troubles

If you are intolerant to gluten, it can affect your skin, too. A symptom and effect of celiac disease known as dermatitis herpetiformis leads to the formation of blisters on the skin. People who have this disease are sensitive to gluten, but at least 10% of these patients have trouble with digestion, which is an indication of celiac disease. There are various skin diseases that you can prevent or overcome when you follow a gluten-free diet. These problems include:

GHz

Psoriasis

This is an inflammatory disease characterized by the reddening and scaling of the skin.

Alopecia Areata

This is an autoimmune disease, a symptom of which is hair loss.

Chronic Urticaria

This condition is characterized by itchy, red, pink, and recurrent lesions with a pale center.

Depression

Over 6% of adults have trouble with depression, and the symptoms vary from one person to the other. Depression can leave you feeling sad or hopeless. People with digestive issues are more prone to developing anxiety and depression than healthy people. These disorders are common among people who have gluten intolerance and celiac disease. There are some theories about gluten intolerance and how it can drive depression. These are:

Fluctuating Serotonin Levels

Your cells use the serotonin neurotransmitter to communicate with each other. This hormone is also known as the happiness hormone, and if your body does not produce enough serotonin, it can cause depression.

Gluten Exorphins

These are peptides that are formed when your body breaks down some gluten proteins. These compounds can interfere with the central nervous system and increase the risk of depression and anxiety.

Changes in the Gut Microbiota

A decrease in beneficial bacteria or an increase in harmful bacteria in the gut can affect your nervous system, increasing the risk of depression and anxiety.

Numerous studies show that people suffering from depression have reported gluten intolerance, and they prefer following a gluten-free diet because it helps them feel better. Their digestive symptoms, however, may not have be resolved. This suggests that exposure to gluten can lead to various digestive symptoms and depression.

Unexplained Weight Loss

Oh yes, this is something you will be happy about, but it is a cause for concern if you lose weight drastically. You can lose weight for different reasons, but one of the most common reasons for unexplained weight loss is celiac disease. A study conducted by Murray A J et al. in 2004 showed that celiac disease patients lose at least two-thirds of their weight before their issue is diagnosed. You can explain this weight loss using different digestive symptoms, and one of the most common reasons is the intestine's inability to absorb food.

Anemia and Iron Deficiency

Anemia is one of the most common issues people face, and this is due to iron deficiency. Over 5% and 2% of American women and men, respectively, have an iron deficiency. The symptoms include fatigue, low blood volume, pale skin, weakness, dizziness, headaches, and shortness of breath.

If you have celiac disease, your small intestine cannot absorb the nutrients from the food you eat. This reduces the iron your body can absorb. Iron deficiency is one of the common symptoms of celiac disease, and this symptom is one that your doctor will notice. Recent research shows that people with celiac disease have iron deficiency.

Anxiety

Anxiety is a mental disorder that affects at least 15% of people across the globe. This disorder involves feelings of nervousness, agitation, unease, and worry. People with gluten intolerance are more prone to panic disorders and anxiety than other individuals. A study conducted by Volta U et al. in 2014 showed that people with gluten sensitivity experience anxiety.

Autoimmune Diseases and Disorders

An example of an autoimmune disease is celiac disease, which causes your immune system to attack your digestive system when you consume gluten.

Having this autoimmune disease makes you prone to developing other immune diseases like autoimmune thyroid disease. You may also develop depressive and emotional disorders because of these autoimmune diseases. This makes celiac disease common in those who have autoimmune diseases, such as autoimmune liver disease, inflammatory bowel disease, and type I diabetes. Having said that, gluten sensitivity is not associated with autoimmune diseases, nutritional deficiencies, and malabsorption.

Muscle and Joint Pain

People may experience muscle and joint pains for a variety of reasons. Experts believe that people with celiac disease have a genetically determined over-excitable and over-sensitive nervous system. Such people have a lower pain threshold, which causes the sensory neurons to activate even at the slightest touch, causing pain in joints and muscles. Exposure to gluten can cause inflammation if you are sensitive or have celiac disease. This inflammation can cause pain in the muscles and joints.

Arm or Leg Numbness

Another symptom of intolerance is neuropathy. This symptom involves a tingling or numbness in your arms and legs. This symptom is common in people who have vitamin B12 deficiency and diabetes. It can also be caused by alcohol consumption and toxicity in your body.

Individuals with gluten intolerance or celiac disease are at risk of experiencing numbness in their legs and arms. Nobody can pinpoint the cause of the symptom, but some experts link this symptom to the presence of specific antibodies in your body.

Brain Fog

Brain fog is a term that refers to being unable to focus and think about anything clearly. People have labeled this symptom as having trouble thinking, experiencing mental fatigue, feeling cloudy, and being forgetful. If you have a foggy mind, it is an indication of gluten intolerance, and this is something that almost 40% of individuals with gluten intolerance show. This symptom is caused by a reaction of some antibodies to gluten, but it is difficult to identify the exact reason.

Gluten Allergy and its Kinds

Given the similar properties of the symptoms of many kinds of gluten intolerance and allergies, it becomes difficult to differentiate between the various types. The types and characteristic symptoms of gluten allergies and intolerance are listed below.

Celiac Disease

There's an entire chapter dedicated to celiac disease later in the book, but to brief you at this point, this is the most common type when it comes to gluten allergies. It is, however, not a real allergy. It's an autoimmune disorder, also known as "celiac sprue."

Your body's abnormal immune response against tissues and substances normally found in your body causes an autoimmune disorder. Avoiding regular consumption of foods containing gluten is the only possible way to treat celiac disease. If you have celiac disease and then consume gluten, your immune system will be triggered by the gluten to attack the small intestine's walls. This results in a process in which the small intestine's lining erodes, a process also referred to as "the commencement of villous atrophy." Not only does this condition affect your digestive system, but it can also cause the manifestation of symptoms in different parts of your body.

Non-Celiac Gluten Sensitivity

Also commonly known as gluten sensitivity, its accurate diagnosis is challenging because people suffering from this sensitivity experience some symptoms similar to those caused by celiac disease. Non-celiac sensitivity is more of an inherent immune response and less like an allergic reaction.

Similar to celiac disease, cutting gluten from your diet entirely is the only way to treat non-celiac sensitivity. Constipation, diarrhea, heartburn, bloating, stomach ache, flatulence, anxiety, headache, brain fog, joint pain, tingling in the arms, fatigue, rashes, fatigue, and eczema are common symptoms.

Dermatitis Herpetiformis

Chances are, when someone mentions "gluten" rash, they are referring to dermatitis herpetiformis. It is a type of skin rash characterized by an incessant, deep itch, which occurs when you consume foods containing gluten.

It is an autoimmune disease and not a true allergy; it is caused by an attack of your immune system triggered by gluten indigestion. Rashes can appear anywhere on the body, but most commonly, they show up on the back of the neck, elbows, buttocks, and knees. To keep these rashes under control and prevent them from aggravating, it is important that you avoid food items containing gluten at all costs.

Other symptoms of dermatitis herpetiformis include itching, purple marks on healing skin, many small pimple-like rashes, skin rash, and bumps on the skin. In this case, itching commences before the bumps appear on the skin.

Gluten Ataxia

This is a rare autoimmune condition in which the immune system ends up attacking the brain and neurological system when the person consumes food items containing gluten. This condition falls under gluten allergies.

People suffering from this condition need to consume foods without gluten. If you are suffering from gluten ataxia and consume foods that contain gluten, your immune system will attack the cerebellum, and that could result in some serious, irreversible damage. In addition, this disorder is rather progressive, and while sufferers will start out by experiencing

Arianna Brooks

small problems in the beginning, it could eventually aggravate into something bigger, leading up to consequential disabilities.

Symptoms of gluten ataxia involve clumsiness, deterioration of proper motor skills, difficulty in swallowing, and slurring of speech. It also causes issues with gait, walking, and coordination. While very few sufferers of gluten ataxia experience gastrointestinal symptoms, some who have been diagnosed with it also have villous atrophy, which is found in patients with celiac disease as well.

Wheat Allergy

This one is a true allergy, and it involves compounds of wheat as a culprit, other than just the gluten protein. Wheat allergy is more commonly found in children than in adults. In most cases, it was found that only wheat needs to be taken out of the picture, while rye and barley can be consumed.

Wheat allergy can also result in anaphylaxis, which is a very harmful systemic allergic reaction that is characterized by coughing, slowing down or speeding up of heartbeat, difficulty swallowing, wheezing, and a drop in blood pressure.

Chapter 2: Gluten-Free Diet – What Is It?

To put it simply, a gluten-free diet is a nourishment regime in which the protein gluten is completely excluded. As previously mentioned, gluten is mainly present in grains like rye, wheat, barley, and triticale.

Primarily, the gluten-free diet was developed to treat a condition known as celiac disease. In people with this disease, the consumption of foods that have quantities of gluten results in the inflammation of the small intestine. As explained in the previous chapter, this can be very dangerous for the body.

A gluten-free diet helps in controlling the symptoms of the disease and further prevents all sorts of complications that may arise.

Purpose of the Gluten-Free Diet

Although the gluten-free diet was developed to control and prevent the symptoms of celiac disease, it can still be effective for a large number of people who may not have celiac disease but who suffer from sensitivity to gluten and in whom the consumption of gluten may result in the emergence of many symptoms related to celiac disease. This condition is known as non-celiac gluten sensitivity.

People who suffer from non-celiac gluten sensitivity may or may not choose to follow a gluten-free diet to control the symptoms that they suffer. However, following a gluten-free diet is necessary for people suffering from celiac disease. If they do not, their lives will be riddled with constant symptoms of the disease, which may lead to further complications!

The gluten-free diet has recently become a rising fad and is also believed to be helpful in losing weight.

Nutritional Quality

Gluten-free diets can be quite a powerhouse of high nutritional value and provide you with all the necessary nutrients for a healthy diet. However, the gluten-free diet that is typically followed in the United States lacks specific nutrients, such as the minerals calcium and iron, the B vitamins niacin, riboflavin, and thiamin, and dietary fiber. In addition, a gluten-free diet, much like most American diets, has the makings of being high in fat, including saturated and trans fats.

There haven't been many studies conducted on a gluten-free diet's nutritional adequacy. So far, in the United States, the diet has been evaluated only by one study. It assessed the consumption of calcium, iron, fiber, and grain food items by adults suffering from celiac disease. As per the findings, among the majority of all the females who participated, the intakes of iron, calcium, grain foods, and dietary fiber were below recommended levels. In fact, only 46% had consumed recommended amounts of fiber, 44% for calcium, and just 31% percent consumed appropriate amounts of iron. However, the results were slightly better for men, but 37% and 12% did not consume recommended amounts of calcium and fiber, respectively.

While it is suggested that all readers be watchful of their diet's nutritional adequacy, it is of utmost importance that women pay extra attention to their consumption of these nutrients.

It is vital that you are armed with enough information on nutrition to avoid the pitfalls when on a gluten-free diet. Here's how:

B Vitamins, Iron, and Dietary Fiber

There are varieties of food categorized as whole-grain and fortified or enriched. These are foods, such as pasta, bread products, and breakfast cereals, which contribute a sizable amount of iron, B vitamins, and dietary fiber to the average American's diet. However, it might be difficult to access these nutrients when you are on a gluten-free diet because the majority of bread products, cereals, and pastas manufactured as gluten-free are neither enriched nor whole-grain.

Foodstuffs that are specially manufactured as gluten-free, such as pastas, cereals, and breads, are mostly made using starches like cornstarch, rice starch, and potato starch or refined flours like milled corn and milled rice. When a grain like brown rice is refined during the milling process to make white rice, the two components that are removed are the germ and bran of the grain, but a lot of the minerals, vitamins, and dietary fiber found in grains come from these very parts.

In the United States, most refined wheat-based pastas and breads undergo a process of voluntary enrichment. They are "enriched" with folic acid (the synthetic form of folate), thiamin, riboflavin, niacin, and iron. Enrichment refers to the nutrients (except fiber) lost during the process of milling, but then put back into the foodstuffs.

Moreover, many regular breakfast foods like cereals are "fortified" with minerals and vitamins. Sadly, most refined food products that are specially manufactured as gluten-free, like pastas, breads, and cereals, are neither fortified nor enriched. For some unknown reason, many gluten-free food product manufacturers don't enrich their products. Maybe the simplest reason here could be that there is no requirement for them to do so because, in the United States, enriching refined wheat-based grain foodstuffs is voluntary, and their gluten-free alternatives are not required to be enriched.

Whole Grains vs. Refined Grains

Whole grains refer to the whole kernel of grain with the germ, endosperm, and bran intact. Refined grains originate from whole grains but undergo processing to attain a finer texture and shelf-life durability. Unfortunately, this process is when the germ and bran are removed. This removal also results in the elimination of iron, dietary fiber, and a lot of B vitamins.

Enriched v. Fortified

There will be many instances when you will come across these terms. They are often used interchangeably when referring to food items, but they are, in fact, not the same. Generally, when you find the term *enriched* on a food label, it refers to the addition of minerals and vitamins back into the refined grain food product that they originally were present in, but were removed from, during the milling process.

Based on the regulations of the Food and Drug Administration, only specific foods in the U.S. can be enriched voluntarily with specific minerals and vitamins. This is done partly for the prevention of overconsumption of a certain nutrient. Food products that may be enriched are flour, buns, rolls, breads, noodle items, rice, farina, and cornmeal, to name a few. However, to be labeled as enriched, these items need to contain specific amounts of thiamin, riboflavin, niacin, iron, and folic acid.

Additionally, foodstuffs may be fortified with a wide range of minerals and vitamins that may not have been present in the original food item. The specified amount of certain nutrients allowed to be added to fortified foods may or may not be regulated, depending on the elaborated nutrient and food. Some examples of fortified foods are soymilk, energy bars, breakfast cereal, and orange juice.

Enriched vs. Unenriched

Enriched and whole-grain food products are more nutritionally dense than unenriched and refined foods. It also means that for the same calorie content, they offer much higher levels of nutrients.

Fat

There are no innate aspects to a gluten-free diet that would make it more or less likely to be high in fat. Even so, most gluten-free diets are indeed high in their recommended quantity of consumption of fat. For overall wellbeing and health, people with celiac disease are suggested to pay extra attention to the fat content in their diet, especially in terms of trans and saturated fats. Any diet that has a lot of processed snack foodstuffs, fatty meat items, and full-fat dairy foods may be very high in unhealthy fat.

Fiber

Yes, gluten-free diets can contain enough amounts of fiber, but it's important to take that extra step to ensure you choose food items that are, in fact, good sources of fiber. Based on studies, most Americans consume half of the recommended intake of dietary fiber.

In fact, in your average American diet, an adult's intake of fiber consists of over 25% of grain foods, such as pasta, flour, ready-to-eat cereals, and yeast breads, to mention a few.

Many gluten-free foods are made from starches and refined flours, components that contain very little amounts of fiber, and as a result, processed grain foods that are a part of a gluten-free diet may not be great sources of fiber.

Including Fiber in Your Diet

All plant foods, such as legumes, whole grains, fruits, and vegetables, contain fiber. While you will see a lot of suggestions to add fiber, a word of caution: it is recommended that fiber be added to your diet at a gradual pace. A quick rise in your fiber intake can result in some problems, such as intestinal and stomach distress, as well as diarrhea, bloating, and gas. These are also conditions that are, now and then, incorrectly associated with a gluten reaction. Nevertheless, when your fiber consumption is increased gradually, the chances of developing these reactions are largely reduced.

Folate

With the right food and dietary choices, a gluten-free diet can offer you enough folate on a regular basis. However, it might not be so easy to consume the recommended quantities of folic acid from enriched food products for someone who follows a gluten-free diet as compared to someone on a regular American diet.

In the U.S., the majority of refined wheat-based bread, flour, breakfast cereals, and pastas are fortified or enriched with folic acid. Given that most refined gluten-free grain products are not enriched, for people following a gluten-free diet, this source of folate is not as readily available.

Including Folate in Your Diet

You can increase your folate intake by consuming various gluten-free food products. These also include food products that naturally contain folate and foods that have been enriched with folate.

Consuming foods enriched with folate is highly essential for women who are capable of becoming pregnant. In case you fall under this category, folic acid is easily absorbed from supplements (gluten-free supplements if you are on the diet) and enriched food products rather than from normal food. Although the majority of manufacturers of gluten-free breads, flours, breakfast cereals, and pastas do not enrich their products, some do.

Iron

Pick your dietary inclusions well, and a gluten-free diet will provide you with enough iron. It is, however, true that someone on a gluten-free diet may find it harder to consume iron than someone on a normal diet. This is especially true for women at the premenopausal stage of their life. Women between the ages of 19 and 50 require twice the amount of iron, as opposed to their male counterparts of similar ages.

In the United States, a third of an adult's intake of iron is accounted for by grain-based food products, mostly as a result of enrichment; many wheat-based grain foods are enriched with iron, while most breakfast cereals are fortified with it.

It is worth mentioning that whole grains are a great and vital source of iron. Most gluten-free products are made from refined starches and flours, so very little iron is present in them.

Including Iron in Your Diet

To increase your consumption of iron, make sure you consume a wide range of gluten-free enriched and whole grains, alongside poultry, legumes, vegetables, lean meat, and fruit.

Calcium

While people with untreated celiac disease might not absorb enough calcium, there is hardly anything about gluten-free diets that would limit calcium intake.

In the typical American diet, the main sources of calcium – milk and cheese – are easily available to people who are following a gluten-free diet. However, it is worth noting that people with celiac disease usually develop a temporary secondary form of intolerance toward lactose and are unable to digest the sugar in milk-based foodstuffs. If you can relate, there are still lots of calcium-containing foods that you can consume.

Including Calcium in Your Diet

If you are lactose intolerant or if you are following a vegan or vegetarian diet, try opting for a diet that's low in fat, or simply avoid consuming dairy products.

Thiamin, Riboflavin, and Niacin

With a bit of effort put into proper meal planning, a gluten-free diet can provide you with sufficient amounts of thiamin, riboflavin, and niacin. In the United States, about 30% of an adult's intake of thiamin, riboflavin, and niacin is accounted for by grain-based foodstuffs. Largely, it is as a result of these foods being enriched with B vitamins.

Including Thiamin, Riboflavin, and Niacin in Your Diet

Instead of leaning toward refined gluten-free foods, try opting for whole-grain gluten-free foods. Some examples of gluten-free whole grains are brown rice, millet, sorghum, wild rice, teff, whole corn flour, whole cornmeal, amaranth, buckwheat, and quinoa.

Moreover, opt for enriched gluten-free grain food products over unenriched and refined varieties whenever you can.

Tips to Make it Easier to Adjust to a Gluten-Free Life

Switching from a regular diet to a gluten-free diet is a very big change, and it will take your body some time to get used to it. In the first few days, you may feel that the diet is very restrictive, and it may be frustrating that you can't even eat more than half the stuff that is in your kitchen or pantry.

The first thing you have to do is to stop thinking about the things you can't eat and instead focus on the things that you can actually eat. Yes, it is easier said than done, but this is the first step you need to take so that you don't relapse and end up eating something that will make you seriously ill. It has become increasingly easy to find gluten-free versions of all your favorite foods and snacks; all you need to do is read the labels!

Another point to keep in mind is to look for specialty gluten-free stores in your area. This way, you will be able to find gluten-free products easily, without the temptation of buying something that contains gluten. If you can't find such products, try contacting your local celiac support group so that they can guide you!

Moreover, during the initial days of following the diet, it is best to talk to a dietician about the switch and take their advice about the easiest way and the best means to get all the nutrients that your body requires without compromising on the diet.

If you live alone, I advise that you get rid of all the food from your kitchen and pantry that does not conform to your diet. You could give the food to a relative or friend, or even donate the food to an orphanage or to the Salvation Army. This will make it easier for you to follow the diet.

When you're out for meals with your family, friends, or business associates, take care that no cross contamination of food occurs. This is because even a single crumb from bread can cause symptoms in your body or elevate existing symptoms to a more serious level. As a rule of thumb, do not share plates or cutlery with anyone. If someone wants a bite off your plate, insist that he or she use fresh cutlery and not the cutlery that they have been using to eat their meal.

If you live with a family member, a partner, or a roommate who does not follow a gluten-free diet, it is advisable that you buy two separate jars of foods like butter, peanut butter, jam, mayonnaise, cream cheese, Nutella, etc., to ensure that no cross contamination occurs.

Moreover, mark gluten-free products with a flashy tape, paint, or even stickers. This will ensure that there is no mix up of gluten-free and gluten-containing products.

In addition, invest in a second set of electronics, like a toaster, to easily toast your delicious gluten-free-bread (that tastes even more delicious after being toasted) and to ensure that there are no gluten-filled crumbs stuck to it. If you don't want to invest in a second toaster, you can toast your bread in the oven – just place it on a piece of aluminum foil or use the special bags that are manufactured for this reason.

Invest in a good cookbook that has various gluten-free versions of your favorite dishes. This will ensure that you do not fall off the wagon and that, when you are craving something in particular, you can make a diet-friendly version of the dish you are craving for instead of just taking the easy way out.

Benefits of the Diet

A gluten-free diet has many benefits, especially if you have a gluten allergy or celiac disease. This section covers some of the benefits of the diet.

Relieves Digestive Symptoms

People who follow a gluten-free diet do not have as many digestive problems as those who do not. Some symptoms of digestive disease include constipation, fatigue, diarrhea, bloating, gas, and other symptoms.

A study conducted in 2004 by Norstrom F et al. concluded that people, especially those with gluten sensitivity or celiac disease, who follow a gluten-free diet do not experience too many digestive issues.

A study conducted by Murray A J et al. in 2004 concluded that people who follow a gluten-free diet for six months do not experience stomach pain. They also do not experience diarrhea and nausea often and do not show any other symptoms.

Reduces Chronic Inflammation

If you have celiac disease, you may have trouble with inflammation. Inflammation is a your body's response to be able to heal and treat an infection. Inflammation can last for a few days or weeks, and in this case, it is called chronic inflammation. This could be because of various health issues, one of which is celiac disease.

If you follow a gluten-free diet, it can help reduce inflammation caused by celiac disease and other allergies. A study conducted in 2004 by Midhagen G et al. concluded that a gluten-free diet can reduce symptoms of inflammation. It can also help you overcome any damage caused to the gut because of gluten-related inflammation.

People who are sensitive to gluten may also have trouble with inflammation. It is not completely clear if a gluten-free diet can reduce the symptoms of inflammation.

It Gives You an Energy Boost

People with gluten allergies or celiac disease feel tired, experience brain fog, and are sluggish. Experts believe that these symptoms arise because of some nutrient deficiencies that damage the gut. For instance, an iron deficiency can lead to anemia, which is a common symptom of celiac disease.

If you have gluten allergies or celiac disease, it is best to switch to a gluten-free diet. This will improve your energy levels and prevent you from feeling sluggish and tired.

A study conducted in 2012 by Norstrom F et al. had 1031 subjects with celiac disease. At the end of the study, it was found that the subjects who followed a gluten-free diet did not experience fatigue.

Aids in Weight Loss

It is not unusual for a person to lose weight when he or she follows a gluten-free diet because this eliminates or reduces junk food consumption. This also reduces the number of unwanted calories in your diet. These foods are replaced by lean proteins, fruit, and vegetables.

Having said that, you need to avoid consuming "gluten-free" foods, such as snacks, cakes, and pastries. These add too many calories to your diet. You need to focus on the consumption of unprocessed and whole foods, such as fruits and vegetables.

Side Effects

There are numerous benefits of a gluten-free diet, but there are also some downsides to it. The following are some negative effects of this diet:

Increased Risk of Nutritional Deficiency

People with celiac disease or gluten allergy are at risk of developing nutritional deficiencies, including iron, fiber, calcium, folate, vitamin B12, vitamins A, D, E, and K, and zinc.

A study conducted in 2016 by Vici G et al. showed that you could not treat nutritional deficiencies if you follow a gluten-free diet. This happens because people on such diets choose processed foods as these are labeled "gluten-free" by manufacturers. They do not consume nutritious foods, such as vegetables and fruits.

Most gluten-free versions of food do not have vitamin B, and they are not fortified with folate. Fortified bread is a good source of vitamins, but if you follow a gluten-free diet, you cannot eat this food. This increases the risk of developing deficiencies. This is especially difficult for pregnant women with gluten allergies or celiac disease because vitamin B is essential for the baby.

Constipation

Constipation is another side effect of a gluten-free diet. As most diets eliminate or reduce your intake of fiber, such as bran, whole wheat products, and bread, your body will find it hard to get rid of waste. Therefore, you need to increase your intake of foods rich in fiber if you want to improve your bowel movements.

Additionally, most gluten-free substitutes of wheat-based products do not have a lot of fiber. This is another reason why it is common for people to feel constipated. If you have trouble with bowel movements when you are on a gluten-free diet, you need to increase your intake of fruits and vegetables, such as beans, broccoli, Brussels sprouts, berries, and lentils.

Cost

It is difficult for you to stick to a gluten-free diet, especially if you are on a tight budget. A study conducted in 2008 by Stevens L and Rashid M concluded that gluten-free foods are almost three times more expensive than regular products.

Gluten-free foods are more expensive for manufacturers to make, and thus, they are more expensive. For instance, gluten-free foods need to pass a strict testing process to ensure they are not contaminated. If you cannot spend as much on a gluten-free diet, you can stick to single-ingredient and whole foods. These cost less.

Socializing Can Become Difficult

As most social situations revolve around eating and conversing, it becomes difficult for you to socialize if you follow a diet. Most restaurants now have gluten-free options, but there is a risk that some of these foods may be contaminated with traces of gluten.

A study conducted in 2008 by Leffler D A et al. concluded that over 22% of people have celiac disease, and they avoid social events and gatherings so they can stick to their diet.

Having said that, you can socialize with a lot of people even when you are following a gluten-free diet. The only thing you need to do is prepare before you step out of the home. For instance, if you are going to eat out, call ahead and check with the restaurant if they have gluten-free options. If you are going to social events, you can carry your own food if you need to.

Arianna Brooks

Chapter 3: Eating Paleo – What Is It and How Does It Work?

Eating Paleo, also known as the caveman diet or the Paleolithic diet, is a diet in which you ingest only the foods that our ancestors may have consumed, such as meats, berries, and nuts, while avoiding the consumption of foods that they would not have eaten, like grains and dairy.

The proponents of eating Paleo claim that during the Paleolithic era – an era in which man was primarily a hunter that lasted for about 2.5 million years – the human body evolved in such a way as to adapt to the nutrition available to them at that time. That is, human nutritional needs adjusted to the foods available to them at that time.

With the advent of agriculture and the domestication of animals, our food started evolving at a rapid pace, and in a mere 10,000 years since the end of the Paleolithic era, we have gone from hunting animals and gathering berries to consuming a wide variety of processed and grown foods.

According to the advocates of Paleo, human metabolism has failed to evolve fast enough and adjust to the rapidly evolving foods that have become available since the Paleolithic age ended. To put it simply, our bodies are not completely equipped to handle the food that we are eating now.

Hence, we have not completely adapted to eating all the foods that we have developed since the end of the Paleolithic era. These foods include dairy products, legumes, grains, and alcohol. A common belief is that the inability of our bodies to properly digest these new foods and absorb the nutrition from them has caused a rise in the occurrence of cardiovascular diseases and a significant increase in the instances of obesity and diabetes.

Furthermore, the proponents of this diet claim that if an individual follows Paleo, he or she will lead a life that is healthier, more active, and longer than that of the people who do not follow the principles of Paleo.

Nutrients That You Consume While Eating Paleo

- **Protein:** It is recommended that protein make up at least 10% to 35% of your total calories because it is believed that protein constituted approximately 19% to 35% of the calories consumed by our Paleolithic ancestors who were on this hunter-gatherer diet. The high consumption of meats and seafood will ensure that you meet this requirement.

- **Carbohydrates:** According to the recommendations for this diet, you should consume fewer carbs, and about 45% to 65% of your total calorie intake should come from non-starchy fruits and vegetables.

- **Fats:** Fats consumed should be monounsaturated fats, polyunsaturated fats, and omega-3 fats. Meanwhile, the consumption of omega-6 fats and trans fats should be completely avoided.

- **Fiber:** Fiber intake from fruits and vegetables should be high to facilitate proper bowel movement.

- **Vitamins:** The consumption of meats, fruits, and vegetables ensures that your body receives vitamins A, B_1, B_2, B_6, C, D, E, and K, as well as folic acid.

- **Calcium:** Despite popular belief, dairy and dairy products are not the sole sources of calcium. Seeds like sesame and chia, vegetable greens like Bok choy and turnip greens, green veggies like broccoli, fruits like figs, nuts like almonds, and seafood like herring are rich, non-dairy, and Paleo-friendly sources of calcium.

Foods You Can Eat

This list contains the foods that are said to have been readily available to cavemen for consumption. This is why, while following Paleo, you are allowed to consume all the foods on this list.

- **Lean Meats** like lamb, beef, pork, veal, and sausages

- **Seafood** like fish, crab, lobster, oyster, clam, octopus, shrimp, and prawns

- **Fruits** like apples, oranges, melons, strawberries, cherries, blueberries, bananas, grapes, etc.

- **Vegetables** like tomatoes, sweet potatoes, cucumbers, zucchini, carrots, peas, broccoli, Bok choy, turnip greens, etc.

- **Nuts** like walnuts, almonds, cashew nuts, peanuts, hazelnuts, Brazil nuts, chestnuts, pecans, candlenut, macadamia nuts, pine nuts, etc.

- **Seeds** like sesame seeds, chia seeds, coriander seeds, mustard seeds, quinoa, etc.

- **Healthy Oils** like coconut oil, olive oil, walnut oil, avocado oil, flaxseed oil, macadamia nut oil, etc.

Foods You Cannot Eat

These foods are said to be unavailable to cavemen. Thus, while following Paleo, you cannot consume any of the foods on this list.

- **Dairy Products** like milk, cheese, curd, cream cheese, butter, buttermilk, cream, condensed milk, ice cream, etc.

- **Grains** like rye, barley, wheat, canary seed, triticale, etc. The exclusion of grains makes this diet gluten-free and ideal for those who do not want to consume gluten.

- **Legumes** like chickpeas, dry beans, fava beans, peas, peanuts, soybeans, yam beans, etc.

- **Processed Oils** like sunflower oil, canola oil, soya bean oil, cottonseed oil, safflower oil, corn oil, etc.

- **Refined Sugar** like that in sodas, jellies, jams, sports drinks, energy drinks, etc.

- **Table Salt**

- **Alcohol** like wine, beer, vodka, whiskey, tequila, etc.

- **All Variants of Coffee**

- **Processed foods** like chips, crackers, pretzels, biscuits, etc.

Habits to Forsake while Following Paleo

Alcohol

- Curbing this habit might prove to be a tad difficult if you're in any way a heavy drinker, but here's the good news –Paleo in no way requires you to stop drinking entirely. If you are following the diet well, you are allowed a specific quantity of alcohol.

- Consuming alcohol, as an indulgence, has become more of a chance to dabble in lighthearted humor and fun with people close to you, instead of just being an excuse to make you fall off your seat.

- After a long and hectic day, having that evening drink in a relaxed atmosphere can sometimes be really good for your health. A lot of us enjoy occasional drinks with our dear ones, but yes, there are those who are into a regular habit of drinking. They drink not only out of habit but also have absolutely no control over their alcohol consumption. If you are one of them, it would help to go off alcohol completely for a few days prior to starting the diet plan. Once you've steadied yourself with the diet, you can let yourself go for an occasional drink – maybe even two.

- If studies are anything to go by, alcohol, in moderate consumption, can affect our health in positive ways, but the mistake most people make as regards alcohol is that they overdose on it, which makes it toxic to their bodies. There may have been many instances where your friends pressured you into having a few more drinks past your drinking limit, and let's face it, it's not difficult to give into their demands. All things considered, if you're eating Paleo, you will have to make sure that you free yourself of this habit. However, if you still want to have a drink now and then, feel free to follow the tips mentioned below to keep you from overdosing on it.

- In the case of attending a party, indulge in a meal that's low in carbs and high in protein beforehand. This works wonders in putting your alcohol craving under control.

- Have some mental preparation at hand. Keep a mental note of the number of drinks you're going to have before you attend a party and make sure you stick to it.

- For every small peg, drink at least one glass of water. Not only will this ensure that your body stays hydrated throughout the entire ordeal, but it will also limit how much you're going to drink.

- Consider ordering something like a club soda and squeeze some fresh lime onto it. What this does is that it works as a vodka impostor and keeps your peers from questioning your sobriety.

- If you end up drinking a bit more, then for the next few days, completely stop your alcohol intake.

Smoking

- This gets an absolute no if you intend to follow Paleo. In case you are unable to get rid of this habit before starting off on Paleo, the diet will help you remove this habit forever. A lot of people have reported developing disgust for the taste of cigarettes just within a few weeks of eating Paleo. While this might sound unbelievable to a lot of people, when you acquaint your body with consuming non-toxic foods, it will, by default, begin rejecting any harmful thing, including cigarettes.

There have even been reports of people getting headaches and feeling nauseous from smoking just one cigarette. As it turns out, quitting smoking while eating Paleo is much easier than expected. Changing your lifestyle for the betterment of your health by following Paleo makes you feel motivated enough to steer clear of habits that are harmful for your health, such as smoking.

Benefits of Eating Paleo

Detox

Detoxing has become an essential ingredient for a lot of people's health regime. The ever-increasing amount of pollution and impurities in the environment have people rushing into diets and plans to cleanse their bodies. Owing to food and ecological carriers, these impurities pervade our system and settle in our bodies.

Arianna Brooks

When you consume huge amounts of foods containing MSG, refined sugar, or caffeine or consume foods loaded with trans fats, some very harmful toxins tend to settle into your body. While eating Paleo, you detoxify your body because you do not consume any type of preservative, chemical, or additive. Given that Paleo primarily involves consuming natural food items, you will, by default, end up bypassing these deleterious additives by letting your body get some much-needed rest.

Eating Paleo strongly promotes the consumption of natural and healthy foods, as only these are capable of detoxifying your body. Fiber, phytonutrients, and antioxidants are abundantly found in natural foods, and these nutrients are crucial for the purgation of all the toxins that accumulated in your body. In addition, they also leave you feeling a lot more active, energized, and light.

Another essential aspect of Paleo is that, unlike most diets, it does not require you to go on any kind of liquid-specific diet to deal with any difficult cravings you might run into. In fact, similar benefits can be reaped while sticking to consuming regular meals.

The Anti-Inflammatory Effect

Many types of food contain allergens, and these can be harmful for a huge part of the population. Milk and grains are two of the food items that most commonly cause allergies, and these two foods are to be avoided at all costs when following Paleo. The nutrients present in vegetables, nuts, fruits, oils, and seeds have an anti-inflammatory effect on your body. To be specific, they help avoid inflammation of the stomach, heart, etc.

Prevention of Disorders and Diseases

Processed foods are one of the major malefactors in the increase in the incidence of diabetes and obesity all around the world. These food items contain many types of harmful components, along with fillers that serve next to no purpose apart from enhancing the taste.

Some chemicals found in different processed food products are so deleterious that they might even lead to a multitude of health problems, such as cancer, pancreatic diseases, cardiac issues, hepatic problems, diabetes, etc. Many processed foodstuffs also contain high amounts of preservatives. Chemicals like butylated hydroxyanisole or BHA and butylated hydroxytoluene or BHT have been proven to affect our neurological system negatively in many ways and are also known to cause cancer.

By eating Paleo, you can bypass all of these chemicals that threaten your health without making any additional effort. It is also worth noting that Paleo foods contain an insanely high number of antioxidants and phytonutrients, which, other than keeping you energized, can also put up a fight against all the aforementioned diseases. As the diet is a rich source of fiber, vitamins, and healthy fats, it results in an overall healthy life for you.

Satiation

For the majority of people, a diet is, by default, synonymous with constant bouts of hunger, and while that is true in the case of most diets, when following Paleo, the chances of feeling any kind of hunger or going to bed with an empty tummy are pretty slim.

As you consume larger quantities of proteins and fats, you feel satiated after each meal, and your "in between meals" are cut down because you don't feel hungry easily. You can even find yourself going without any cravings throughout the day. This is what consuming the proper amount of fruit, vegetables, and meats in every meal does for your body; it easily enables you to go about your day without feeling any hunger in the first place.

Weight Loss

One of the most sought-after benefits and attractions of diets is weight reduction. What makes eating Paleo specifically effective in this context is that you'll be losing weight in no time once you start following the diet. Paleo's supposition of consuming only natural foods while on the diet and the stark reduction in the consumption of processed and unnatural foods lays the foundation here as the lack of refined sugars, trans fats, and high glycemic carbohydrates in this diet can help you lose weight a lot faster.

One of the aspects that make Paleo an effortless method for losing weight that is so easy to follow is that you face no need to put a stop to your eating or the incessant requirement to measure every calorie that enters your body. Unlike most diets that demand you to keep a mathematical track of each and every calorie in every bite of your food, Paleo lets you forsake all reigns as regards eating whatever you want, as long as it is within the guidelines of the diet. This liberty frees you from the unwieldy process of attempting a diet and lets you follow something so easy to work with.

After being on Paleo for some time, you start getting the hang of it, and soon enough, you'll find yourself enjoying the entire process that you might even forget that you're on a diet! Throughout all of this, you'll be consistently losing weight! The fun factors of the diet don't let you look at it from a miserable perspective, and this, in turn, is highly rewarding as it makes sure you'll be sticking to the diet and avoiding whatever resentment was previously possible.

Goodbye, Calorie Calculations

As mentioned above, one of the most tiresome and cumbersome activities is calculating your calorie intake – to measure and account for all the calories you've consumed and subsequently burned. Most diets hand you calorie charts and calculators so that your calorie consumption doesn't exceed the specified amount. However, Paleo eliminates such headaches and ensures you're not haunted by the ghosts of math. This diet is extremely easy to follow because you don't need to measure every portion size or every calorie that you consume.

Better Sleep Cycles

Sleep is one of the most essential needs of any and every living creature. While we do not know a lot about sleep, what we do know is that it holds extreme importance, and irregular or uncomfortable sleeping cycles can be the stuff of nightmares.

Processed foods often contain chemicals like caffeine and many others, which have a tendency to obstruct our natural sleeping patterns and lead to sleep discomfort. A natural compound called serotonin, which is released by our brain to make us sleepy, often gets overridden by additives from processed food. However, following Paleo and depending on natural foods and compounds make us sleep better. Not only does it improve the quality of our sleep but it also prompts our body into feeling energized and pumped just a few days after starting to eat Paleo. This is one of the signs that your body is synchronizing itself with the natural circadian cycle, much like our ancestors.

Cutting Down on Junk Consumption

In today's world, "time is of the essence" has never been so stressed upon as before. The rushed schedule people are trying to keep up with has all the aspects of their life bound by time constraints. This franticness vastly affects your dietary habits as well, where, like most people, you'll find yourself depending on unrestricted amounts of fast food or junk food items that are highly disadvantageous for your health. All of this dependence on junk food results from just trying to satisfy your hunger.

It is a well-established fact that these unhealthy foods come with little to almost no nutrients essential for the body; instead, they're a package of artificial chemicals constantly attacking your system. Being on Paleo steers you clear of junk foods and saves your body from high cholesterol and other disorders detrimental to your health. Another factor associated with this point is that you start saving a fair amount of money that you'd generally spent on fast food, etc.

Instead, you can divert those expenses toward something that is so beneficial for your body, from buying organic foods to Paleo books, all of which will help you on your Paleo journey. Cutting down on junk and fast food can prove to be very difficult for most individuals in the beginning because it's not only an adjustment made on a psychological level but also on a physical level, and that goes to show to what extent these foods have entrapped our diet.

For instance, there are brands of cookies that are nearly as addictive as cocaine or morphine. They're better at activating the pleasure centers in our brain much more effectively than most drugs. This also stands true in the case of French fries and potato chips. However, with a bit of effort and dedication, you can overcome such substances with a lot of ease.

Increased Energy Levels

Paleo is abundant in naturally produced fruit, roots, and vegetables. When paired properly, a Paleo meal can have the right balance of proteins, vitamins, carbs, minerals, and all essential nutrients. The high protein and low carbohydrate content of the diet makes you feel energetic, such that you do not experience any lethargy.

Healthier Body Cells, Healthier Brain

The human body is built of an innumerable number of cells, and these cells consist of unsaturated and saturated fats. The health of a cell entirely depends on the perfect balance between these two fats. Paleo is one of those diets that effectively help your body maintain that balance, as you're supposed to consume both types of fats while on the diet. This is unlike most diets where your expected consumption of fats is restricted to only one kind. Apart from that, eating Paleo is highly beneficial for the health of your nervous system and brain.

For anyone who wants to be on Paleo, salmon is one of the highly recommended food items; it's rich in omega-3 fatty acids that are often, for the most part, lacking in the average American person's regular diet. Omega-3 comes with a high amount of DHA, a compound that is vital for the body and growth of the brain, heart, and eyes. It's also found in pasture-grown meats and eggs.

Helps Maintain Blood Glucose Levels

Saying we are indeed living in an age dominated by sugar would most definitely not be a hyperbole. Nearly every other food product we consume has a large amount of sugar in obvious or unobvious forms.

Our monthly intake of sugar is so high that the blood glucose levels of many individuals often fluctuate. However, while eating Paleo, as you practically start cutting off on every sugar-rich food, you very effectively help your body maintain and balance your blood glucose levels. You won't even get tired as a result of sugar crashes that used to occur frequently.

If you're trying to steer clear of diabetes, then this is the most effective diet for you. However, if you're already suffering from diabetes, then it is advisable that you consult your physician before you begin this diet.

There is a marked increase in the intake of iron owing to the consumption of red meats.

Drawbacks of Eating Paleo

- Following Paleo can be slightly expensive because you need to purchase organic grass-fed meats, organic fruits and vegetables, and gluten-free versions of all sauces and condiments.

- The non-consumption of dairy can significantly affect the health of your bones if you do not ensure that you are consuming enough calcium-rich foods.

- This diet is extremely difficult for vegetarians to follow, owing to the non-consumption of grains and legumes, which are the two staples for every vegetarian.

- Although this diet plan relies heavily on the consumption of meat, a lot of us don't realize that the meat consumed by our Paleolithic ancestors was a lot leaner than the meat available today. Today, the meat we consume comes from domesticated farm animals that are often stuffed with fodder and often do not leave the confines of their pen, resulting in a large amount of fat deposits on the meat.

- Eating Paleo is slightly lacking in terms of certain micronutrients, such as vitamins B12 and D.

- The "no fixed portion size" makes it very difficult to ensure that you are not overindulging. One bowl of lettuce may not be a problem, but one bowl of nuts may be!

It is difficult to resist cheating because of the strictness of the diet. You can stay consistent for days or even weeks, but consistently following the diet for a few months may be very difficult and may require a great deal of self-control.

Paleo vs. Gluten-Free

Very often, the terms "gluten-free" and "Paleo" are used interchangeably, and many assume that the two are synonymous lifestyles. They are not. You may well be following a gluten-free diet but not a Paleo diet, or vice versa, and it is important to understand what the differences are and how they can tie in with one another.

For many people, cutting gluten out of their diet is the first stage in making their lives healthier, and yes, there are some great reasons why a gluten-free diet is the way to go; you will almost certainly notice a difference in how healthy you feel and how much more energy you have.

Gluten sensitivity is estimated to affect around 18 million people in the U.S. alone, yet it remains one of the primary parts of the standard American diet. The last 10 years or so have been quite enlightening in terms of information that helps doctors understand the links between gluten and inflammation, and this is what kick-started the gluten-free trend.

Yes, you can find gluten-free products in the stores – there's a whole range of cookies, chips, pancakes, donuts, waffles, brownies, and much more. However, following a gluten-free lifestyle doesn't mean that you can still eat these foods; they are highly processed, packed with sugar, salt, artificial sweeteners, chemicals, and lots of other stuff that simply isn't good for you.

These gluten-free products may well be part of one of the biggest food industries but, by thinking it's okay to eat them, you are inviting a whole host of other health issues.

What About Paleo?

Incorporating Paleo with a gluten-free style is where you want to be if you want to achieve optimum health. Although a product may say it is gluten-free, it is still full of other rubbish that you really don't want to be putting in your body. So, what you need to do is follow the gluten-free restrictions but also incorporate Paleo principles, keeping away from processed foods and reaping the health benefits in these ways:

- Lower risk of diabetes

- Balanced blood sugar levels

- Lower risk of heart disease

- Lower risk of some cancers

- Clearer skin

- Higher energy levels

- Significantly improved digestion

- Much healthier hair

- Much lower risk of chronic inflammation

The Paleo lifestyle is focused on consuming non-inflammatory foods, thus providing a stronger foundation for optimum health. Most chronic conditions we live with today are related directly to inflammation in the body, and when you can lower this, more often than not, those chronic conditions disappear.

Why is Gluten So Bad?

When you follow a Paleo lifestyle, you are not allowed to consume any grains – take up Paleo, and, straight away, you are living a gluten-free life. Gluten is a wheat protein that helps nourish the plant while it germinates and grows, but it can also be found in other grains, such as rye, barley, and many cross-bred grains. After grinding and being used for baking, gluten changes the texture of baked goods, and this is why many people prefer to use wheat and other grains for baking purposes.

Not everyone can tolerate gluten, and their immune response may be abnormal when they consume it. Sometimes, the response may happen immediately after eating and will be noticeable, while other times, the response may not be that noticeable. This is why many people continue to consume gluten, not realizing the havoc it is wreaking in their health.

In fact, most people who are intolerant continue to eat it daily, and the health issues creep up on them. Lack of energy, indigestion, and general aches and pains are all caused by inflammation. You may not make the association between gluten and your health, but when you stop consuming it, you will certainly notice a significant decrease in your symptoms.

The biggest reason why there are so many gluten-intolerant people in the world today is that wheat has changed beyond all recognition over the years. Using modern technology, scientists like nothing more than to play god and change the wheat, such that the wheat you eat today is around 80% gluten.

What Else Does Paleo Eliminate?

Given that Paleo eliminates grains, it also eliminates two other compounds that contribute to poor digestion and chronic inflammation. Alongside gluten, those compounds are:

- **Phytates** – these prevent nutrients from being absorbed by the body by binding with dietary minerals. Phytates are not as harmful as gluten, but you should avoid them as much as you can.

- **Lectins** – small compounds that, when consumed, begin bio-accumulating in the body and damage the gut lining. They can also negatively impact hunger signals, which causes many people to overeat.

Following a Paleo lifestyle will help you avoid these compounds, along with gluten, but if you are only following a gluten-free lifestyle and still consuming processed foods, you are likely still eating them.

The answer? If you want to be truly gluten-free and eliminate inflammation from your body, go Paleo.

Arianna Brooks

Chapter 4: Mistakes to Steer Clear of While Eating Paleo

The Fear of Fats

If conventional ideologies regarding nutrients are anything to go by, the one surrounding fats has to be the most prevalent. We grow up with the idea of fats having only one property, and that's an extension of the word itself. Fattening. Fat. Fats are fattening, obviously! Or are they?

There are a lot – and seriously, a lot – of people who are struck by panic the moment they learn of the absolute presence of fats while following Paleo. That panic naturally evolves into doubt and apprehension regarding the diet's workability, but trust me on this; fats do not equal an increase in weight. This general perception of fats is more misconception than true information. It is, however, important to note that having some facts at hand surely helps in better understanding the role fats play in a diet.

Contrary to very popular beliefs, our bodies are indeed a lot more capable of handling fats than we give them credit for. However, this in no way implies we are supposed to load up on slabs of butter every day and spend no energy on any activity to burn those calories off.

Dietary fat is very fulfilling; it keeps you satiated and is delicious. In fact, the fats stored in our body are where we get our everyday energy to successfully engage in our daily activities. So, how is it possible to antagonize fats without looking at everything fats do for us?

If you ever thought fats do not provide you with any nutritional value, here are some facts for you:

- Fats are an abundant source of vitamin E, a substantial source of choline, high vitamin D, and vitamin K2.

- Our brains require enough fat and glucose to function properly.

- A diet that is high in fat works to prevent brain fog during those times when you end up skipping lunch because you were caught up with work.

- Fats help you lose body fat by enhancing your metabolism, cutting down your incessant cravings, and balancing out your hormones.

Not Being Careful While Shopping

It is not too difficult to get swayed by pretty-looking packaging or products that claim to be "100% natural." However, the obvious needs to be pointed out, and that is, although they come with labels that read "natural," some important Paleo ingredients may be missing from these products, or even worse, they could be full of non-Paleo ingredients. Instead, to be eating Paleo and for it to work, being a smart shopper and reading the labels carefully before buying any product are of extreme importance.

Here are some tips to guide you in being a smart shopper:

Avoid Anything with Excessive Amounts of Sugar in it.

This is one of the most common mistakes followers of Paleo make. That fruit juice you bought, thinking it is completely harmless – did you check the amount of sugar in it? Scary once you think about it, right? Sugar is something that can pretty much ambush you. It can be hidden in canned veggies, condiments, salad dressings, and so on. The only thing you need to do stay careful is check the sugar percentage in the ingredients and then decide whether it is worth buying or not.

Unfamiliar Preservatives or Additives Are Like Strangers You Shouldn't Talk to.

There exists a large variety of additives or preservatives that, in the long run, can be pretty harmful for our health. This is something not a lot of us are aware of. A lot of ingredients we tend to pick up from the supermarket are full of these. For example, it is common knowledge that sodium nitrate is used for preserving meats, and monosodium glutamate is used for the purpose of enhancing the flavor of a food item. However, did you know that it is absolutely *not* okay to use them? Using such products regularly can, in many ways, have links to severe illnesses, such as cancer or ever some chronic diseases. It is best to stay away from these at all costs.

If It Can't Be Classified as Food, Don't Buy It!

It is probably obvious what is being referred to here. All of us are familiar with the temptation of wanting to pick up that fancy-looking or new-to-the-market pretty little packet that gives off the vibes of some food from a far-off magical land or something. Beware! If you pick up something, and it seems to contain all sorts of complicated ingredients that you have difficulty identifying, just put it down and move to the next aisle. If it cannot be categorized as food, are you sure you want to be ingesting it when you're making all these efforts to lead a healthy life with a healthy body? Regardless of how impressive the packaging is, if it doesn't seem like real food, there is not a good enough reason to purchase it.

All or None Mindset

Avoid developing a purist attitude toward your diet; on the occasion you stray from your diet, don't let the failure deter you from getting back on track. It is important to maintain some discipline when you are following Paleo, but you having that one cheat meal does not imply you have completely ruined it all.

When you start off on a diet and make every possible effort to stick to it, it becomes fairly easy to become borderline obsessed with it. The problem with this is that instead of letting the diet cleanse your mind and body into relaxation, you are creating scenarios that will induce a lot of stress in the future. What I mean is that if you fret over the smallest of things to stick to your diet and develop a fear of falling off track, when you do indeed fall off track, chances are you will get stressed out about it. Be disciplined, but also maintain some leniency.

Moreover, there is no need to starve yourself at social gatherings because of the lack of Paleo foods. A lot of those following Paleo find it helpful to simply show up at parties with their own meal, and sometimes, they carry a bit extra to share with their friends and flaunt the benefits of Paleo.

It would be recommended that you stick to an 80/20 regime before going a full 100 or simply to maintain some mental peace about your diet. Notably, 80% of the time, stick strictly to Paleo-specific foods, and the other 20% of the time, let yourself grab some non-Paleo foods. This is a great way to ease into the Paleo routine. However, this should in no way be an excuse to not do a 100% Paleo. Take your time, but do attain it.

Being Under-Prepared

You need to set goals that give you an ample amount of time to prepare yourself before you venture into eating Paleo. Your preparedness will vastly impact the first few weeks and how well you stick to it.

If you are in the middle of the month, be realistic, and instead of going all "I'm going Paleo from tomorrow!" – sit down. Think. Take a piece of paper, or open some note-writing app on your phone, and arrange everything you'll need to do to start your diet. If it's the middle or the end of the month, it would be better if you start the diet from the first week of the next month.

- This helps you keep a calculated track of when you started your diet, how long it has been, etc.

- You can arrange your shopping lists and finish up or get rid of your non-Paleo ingredients until you buy groceries for the next month or the beginning of your Paleo week.

- You can learn everything you need to know to successfully follow Paleo.

Not Preparing Yourself Against Cravings

An established method of curbing non-Paleo cravings would be to go through as many recipes as possible. Knowing how to cook your own meals should be the first priority when going for any diet at all. When you don't have to depend on others or packaged foods for your diet, you exercise a great deal of control over your health.

Every time you want to snack on something, and you are subconsciously leaning toward non-Paleo foods, don't. As mentioned earlier, the occasional non-Paleo cheat meal is okay. However, if you are a sufferer of frequent cravings during your initial weeks, opt for Paleo recipes. There are many recipes that could not only save you from derailing your diet, but these will also come in handy when you need to whip up a quick fix or a meal, be it for yourself or a house party in which you want to treat your friends to homemade Paleo food. Who knows, maybe it will tempt someone into joining in on your Paleo journey. Having others you can discuss Paleo-related things with acts as a great source of encouragement.

No Portion Control

It is commonly mistaken that being on a Paleo means running wild and free with indulgence. Do you think you could hog up on large quantities of meats, butter, poultry, nuts, and everything that tastes divine? Well, no. Let's be rational here for a moment. Gobbling up food like that will only lead to problems, such as gaining weight, etc. It is easy to commit the mistake of not being in control, but fret not; you are most likely not alone in this.

When people learn that eating Paleo allows them to consume whatever food they want to consume, they immediately overdo every single thing.

However, ***consideration is more important than calculation***. Yes, you do not need to calculate your calories, but that in no way implies that you can consume innumerable amounts of them.

There being no portion control is a myth. It exists in every kind of diet, and it is a requirement for you to follow it when on Paleo as well.

Try observing your own eating habits. Do you binge eat when you are stressed? Does your food intake increase during depressing times of your life? These are some things you should be aware of before you begin on your diet plan. Observe them to figure out the exact reason. Every time you feel low or, for some reason, are leaning toward eating to compensate for what you are feeling, tell yourself that this is a habit you need to break away from.

As eating foods rich in fats is allowed in Paleo, it is essential you don't over indulge in them to the point where it creates issues for your body.

When you have just prepared a Paleo meal and crave it immediately, try eating only a bit of it and then some more after a couple of hours. You could also opt for some soup before a meal as a way of indulgence. In this way, you will prevent yourself from eating too much.

No Proper Planning

If you thought eating Paleo could be pulled off without proper planning, think again. Just like every other aspect of our lives that we want to do well in, a diet is no different. To execute it correctly and have the right approach to do so, planning is essential as it builds the base framework of the entire diet and how you should go about it.

If you are someone with a bit of experience with trying this diet or know someone who has, you must be familiar with the importance of getting things organized. In fact, when diets prompt you to organize some things surrounding, say, your food habits or everyday routine, that little nudge to make those small changes goes a very long way.

From identifying Paleo-specific foods and ingredients to checking out farmer's markets to buy meats that are grass-fed, these are small but significant steps that you can take. As mentioned in another section, shop smartly, and be aware of the labels.

If you are plagued by a hectic schedule, plan your meal ahead of time, purchase your Paleo ingredients over the weekend, and store them in the refrigerator. Be sure to wrap your foods appropriately, either with aluminum foil or cling film.

If you are someone who gets bored easily, and even if you are not, eliminate every chance of monotony from your everyday meals. Experiment! Have fun with your food. The possibilities are endless; all you need to do is explore.

Combine ease of cooking and taste. Things become easier to handle if you are making something delicious that does not require a mountain of effort to make.

When you are making breakfast, make sure it is simple but delicious. As for experimentation, do that when you have some extra time on your hands.

One of the flexible characteristics of following Paleo is that it is okay to have leftovers as well. Avoid going overboard with that by having something you made decades ago.

Arianna Brooks

Chapter 5: Tips on Gearing Up While Eating Paleo and Workout Regime

Consuming "real foods" like fruits, vegetables, and meat instead of loading up on dairy, legumes, or even packaged foods works wonders for your body and mind in unimaginable ways. To successfully follow Paleo, there are certain hacks you should have up your sleeve. Sure, there will be a plethora of things you will learn during your experience with Paleo, other than the ones specified below. However, to give you a little nudge toward the starting point, here are some very helpful tips that will help you stay on your Paleo path:

Kitchen Cleansing

Assess your kitchen thoroughly before you go out to buy ingredients specific to your diet. Do non-Paleo ingredients dominate your kitchen? Are you spotting colas, legumes, packaged milk, yogurt, grains, and cereals in your larder? If the answer is yes, it's time to part with these food items and ingredients.

Now, the question arises: What do you do with them? Get rid of them. Simple. Throw them away, or better yet, give them to someone else. However, as being against wastage is the way to go, I'd suggest you give them away to the homeless. You could even donate them to community food centers; if there's anything canned, drop it off at a food bank. Avoid temptations, and any urge to give in to dietary distractions becomes a breeze when the food items and ingredients are miles away from your sight.

Your home and kitchen are places where you are in absolute control of your diet and food consumption. Making these small efforts will benefit you in many big ways in the long run as you eliminate chances of straying from your diet.

Nevertheless, if you're someone who'd like to take it slow instead of turning to such drastic measures, simply start getting rid of non-Paleo foods and ingredients at a much slower pace. Another way to do this would be to wait until your weekly or monthly grocery shopping routine before you start on the diet. This way, you stock up only on the ingredients you will need for the diet and not restock on ingredients strictly prohibited from it.

Goal Setting

Setting goals before starting the diet is a great way to keep yourself motivated and right on track. When trying to lose weight through a diet plan, planning is the key to success. It would also be helpful to contact your physician and check how your body is responding while on the diet. Consulting your physician would be the wise thing to do if you are suffering from chronic illnesses like high blood pressure or even diabetes.

Make sure the goals you set for yourself are realistic. As a start, for the span of a week, just focus on removing non-Paleo foods and ingredients from your kitchen. The next week, aim for a minor milestone as regards your weight loss. Then, as you start progressing, expand and grow the extent of your milestones and aims.

In any scenario, when you fall off track, just make sure you get back to the diet regime without fussing over your derailment. To motivate you on your journey a bit more, you can also share your diet goals on social media or just with your friends; this acts as a nudge compelling you to stick to the diet plan.

Treat Yourself

Every time you successfully reach a goal you have set, reward yourself with something you like. It is just as significant to celebrate your small achievements, as it is to rejoice when meeting the bigger goals. Strike a deal with yourself. Every time you shed a pound, buy yourself a new pair of socks or that other new fancy shampoo you were eyeing at the supermarket. You can even treat yourself to a spa you like, or buy cosmetics you've been thinking of buying but didn't have an incentive to. These small things will motivate you and help you stick to the diet.

The desire to be appreciated and rewarded is pure human nature, and rewards always play the role of apt encouragement for us to happily carry on.

Get a Partner

Ask around your social circles – your friends and colleagues – if anyone would be interested in joining you in enjoying your Paleo regime. Partner workouts are great and effective methods of ensuring you stay on track with your diet; see if you can make time for such partner activities. Following diet plans all by yourself can easily become very boring. It's essential that you enjoy yourself when you are following your diet.

You can also share your everyday progress with your partner; other than just working out together, sharing worthy tips only nudges you forward in the direction of achieving your goals faster than you originally planned on or expected to.

Chapter 6: How to Read Food Labels

When you choose to lead a healthy lifestyle, you must choose the right foods to eat. This does not mean you only need to eat the food you make at home. You can purchase some packaged foods, but you need to read the labels to purchase the right products. Not many people are aware of how to read these labels, so we will discuss the basics and some tips you need to bear in mind when it comes to reading labels.

The Basics of Reading Food Labels

In this section, we will look at the steps you need to follow when reading food labels.

Step One: Understanding the Serving Size

The first thing you need to do is to look for the serving size of the product, which is the amount a person can eat in one go. You also need to look at the total number of servings you can eat. The next thing you need to do is compare the portion size you eat to the serving size listed on the box. It is important to understand that the serving size written on the box applies to the nutrition facts. This means that if one cup of the product is one serving size and you eat two cups, you are eating twice the number of calories, nutrients, and fats than the information listed on the label.

Step Two: Calculate the Total Calories

You need to calculate the total number of calories you consume in one serving based on the ingredients mentioned in the list.

Step Three: Use the Percent Daily Values as a Guide

You need to look at the percent daily values to evaluate and determine the different foods you can regularly consume. You need to check the daily values and see how they will fit into your diet plan. The daily percentage values are for the entire day and not for only one meal. These percentages are the average nutrient levels for a person who eats at least 2,000 calories every day. For example, if the food you eat has 5% fats, it indicates you are consuming 5% of the total fat you can consume throughout the day.

Depending on your goals, you may need to eat more or less than the required daily caloric intake. For some nutrients, you need to eat more or less than the required daily value. If you need to increase your intake of nutrients, increase it only by 20%. You need to increase your consumption of fiber, vitamins, and minerals. If you need to decrease your intake, you need to reduce your intake by 5%.

Step Four: Understand the Nutrition Terms

The following are some terms you need to remember:

- **Low Cholesterol**: This indicates that the food contains 20 milligrams or less of saturated fats in every serving

- **Low Calorie:** This term indicates the food only has 40 calories per serving.

- **Reduced:** If you see this term on a product, it indicates the food has 25% fewer calories and nutrients than the usual.

- **Good source of:** This term indicates that the product provides at least 15% of the required daily value of a particular nutrient or vitamin per serving.

- **High In:** This term indicates the product has 20% more of a nutrient per serving than the required daily value.

- **Calorie-Free**: If you find this term on your product, you need to know it means there are at least 5 calories per serving. Do not fool yourself into thinking the product has no calories.

- **Low Sodium:** This indicates you consume 140 milligrams of sodium with every serving you eat.

- **Sugar-Free/Fat-Free:** This indicates you eat less than ½ a gram of sugar or fat with every serving you eat.

- **Excellent Source of:** This means the product provides at least 20% of the percent daily value of the specified nutrient per serving.

Step Five: Choose Foods Low in Added Sugars, Sodium, and Saturated Fats

When you eat fewer added sugars, as well as less sodium and saturated fats, it reduces the risk of developing chronic heart disease. Trans fats and saturated fats are closely linked to heart diseases, and if you eat too much added sugar, it becomes difficult for you to stick to your daily caloric requirement. Meanwhile, if you increase your sodium intake, it can increase your blood pressure. It is important to remember to decrease your intake of these nutrients to reduce the risk of developing various chronic conditions.

Step Six: Consume Enough Minerals, Fiber, and Vitamins

You need to increase your intake of vitamin D, potassium, iron, fiber, and calcium. You also need to keep yourself active because this reduces the risk of developing health problems, such as anemia and osteoporosis. It is best to add more fruits and vegetables to your diet, especially if you want to increase your nutrient intake. Ensure you consume more nutrients in your diet.

Step Seven: Consider the Other Nutrients

You know about your caloric intake, but it is also important for you to know about the different nutrients present on the label.

Protein

The food label does not indicate the required daily value of protein you need to consume. You need to know how much protein your body needs regularly. Based on your requirements, you need to eat moderate portions of eggs, poultry, yogurt, cheese, lean meat, and low-fat milk. You also need to include peanut butter, peas, beans, soy products, nuts, and seeds.

Carbohydrates

Fiber, sugar, and starch are the three types of carbohydrates, and it is important to limit your intake to ensure you do not develop any chronic diseases. You can eat rice, pasta, fruits, vegetables, cereals, and whole-grain bread.

Sugars

Sugars are simple carbohydrates present in food, such as milk (lactose) and fruit (fructose). These sugars may also come from refined sources, such as corn syrup or sucrose (table sugar). The nutrition label comes with a list of added sugars, too. The 2020–2025 Dietary Guidelines for Americans recommends that you do not consume more than 10% of your daily caloric intake from added sugars.

Foods with more than one ingredient need to have a list on the label. These ingredients are listed in order of weight. The ingredients with the largest amount are listed on top of the list. This information is helpful, especially for someone who has food sensitivities.

Understanding the Process

Most people look at a food label for different reasons, but whatever the reason is, you need to know how to use this information easily and effectively. This section will look at how you can read the labels to enable you to use the stated facts to make informed and quick decisions. This is the only way you can follow a healthy diet.

The information on the top or main section of the nutrition label can vary for every beverage and food product. The label contains specific information about the product, such as calories, nutrient information, and serving size. The bottom section of the label will have footnotes that explain the percent daily value and the number of calories you need to consume to stick to your dietary needs.

Serving Information

When you look at the nutrition label on any product, the first thing you need to do is look at the number of servings on the package. You also need to look at the serving size. These sizes are standardized, thus making it easier for you to compare different products.

The sizes are often provided in common units, such as pieces or cups, along with the metric amount for each size. This metric amount is often in grams. The serving size is an indication of how much a person would typically drink or eat. It is not a recommendation of the quantity you need to drink or eat.

You need to realize that the nutrient amounts on the label, including the number of calories you eat, refer to the servings. You should pay attention to the serving size on the food package to know how much you can eat. Let us assume you want to consume only half a serving of the package. You can use the values on the label to help you calculate this.

For example, the label can state that one serving of a product is equal to one cup of the food. If you eat two cups, that would be two servings. This is twice the nutrients and calories you will consume, as well as the percent daily values.

Calories

The nutrition label indicates the calories consumed per serving.

The number of calories on a label indicates the energy you get when you consume one serving of this food.For example, a label can indicate that one serving of lasagna will provide 280 calories. So, what do you think will happen when you eat the entire package? If the label indicates that a package has four servings, this means you consume 1120 calories.

If you want to maintain or achieve a healthy body weight, you need to balance your caloric intake by watching the food you eat or drink. Your body uses 2,000 calories a day, and this is the required caloric intake for every individual. Having said that, this number will vary for people who need to eat more or less depending on their weight, sex, physical activity, and height. It is important to note the number of servings you consume so you know how many calories you eat each day. If you overeat, then you will gain too much weight or become obese.

Nutrients

A nutrition label should have the list of nutrients, along with their required daily percentage value.

A label will show you the different nutrients present in the product. Using this information, you can determine how the nutrients will impact your health. Use the label to help you meet your dietary needs. If you know what your body needs, look for foods with more of the nutrients your body needs and less of the nutrients you should avoid.

Nutrients to Limit

You need to limit your intake of added sugars, sodium, and saturated fat, which are associated with chronic health issues. These are listed on a nutrition label. Americans often eat large quantities of these foods and cannot stick to the limits.

The American Dietary Association states that you need to consume less of these nutrients. If you eat too much sodium and saturated fat, you can develop various health conditions, such as high blood pressure and cardiovascular disease. If you eat too much sugar, it will become impossible for you to stick to your calorie limits. You also cannot meet your nutrient needs.

Difference Between Added Sugars and Total Sugars

The total sugar on a nutrition label includes the naturally occurring sugars present in nutritious beverages and foods, such as milk, fruit, and vegetables, as well as any added sugar. There is no daily reference value established for the total sugars you can consume because experts could not recommend the total quantity of sugars you can eat every day.

Added sugars on a nutrition label include sugars that were added to the product. These could be added during packaging, such as table sugar, or during food processing, such as dextrose or sucrose. Added sugars also include the sugar in concentrated vegetable or fruit juices, honey, and syrups. If you eat too much sugar, your caloric intake will increase, and it will be difficult for you to stick to your caloric limits.

If the manufacturer puts the word "includes" before the entry for added sugars, it indicates that the grams of total sugars include the number of grams of added sugars.

For example, a container of yogurt may have 8 grams of naturally occurring sugars and 7 grams of added sugars, resulting in a total of 15 grams of sugar.

Nutrients to Eat More of

If you want to lead a healthy lifestyle, you need to increase your intake of vitamin D, iron, calcium, potassium, and dietary fiber. These are the nutrients that most Americans do not get enough of. Thus, you need to ensure that you consume more of these nutrients.

When you follow a diet that is high in dietary fiber, it can ease your bowel movements, lower your cholesterol and blood sugar levels, and reduce your caloric intake. Diets rich in calcium, potassium, iron, and vitamin D can reduce the risk of anemia, high blood pressure, and osteoporosis.

You should use nutrition labels to support your dietary needs and choose the foods that align with your dietary patterns. You also need to purchase foods that contain more nutrients you want to eat and less of those you want to limit.

Understanding the Percent Daily Value

The percent daily value is the percentage of each nutrient that is present in food. These values are based on reference amounts, which are expressed in micrograms, milligrams, and grams of nutrients. This number is an indication of the quantity you cannot exceed per day. The value will show what percentage of a nutrient is present per serving of the food and its contribution to your daily diet. The percentage value will help you determine whether one serving of food has a higher or lower proportion of a specific nutrient.

Does this mean you need to understand how to calculate the percentage daily value? Well, no, because the label has already done the math. You can use the numbers to interpret the number of nutrients per serving and put them on the same scale. If you calculate the sum of the percent daily values in the label, it will not amount to 100%. The daily value of a nutrient is based on one serving of the food you are purchasing. You can use this amount to determine whether the food serving is low or high in a specific nutrient. You can also determine whether one serving of food will contribute to a little or a lot of the nutrients you want to consume.

It is important to note that some nutrients on labels, such as trans-fat and total sugars, do not have a daily value percentage, but we will discuss these later.

General Guide

The following are points to remember when you read the daily percentage value of nutrients:

- If the daily value is 5% or less for a nutrient, it indicates that the nutrient per serving is low.

- If the value is 20% or more, it indicates the serving is high.

You need to choose foods which have a:

- Higher daily value for vitamin D, dietary fiber, potassium, calcium, and iron

- Lower daily value for sodium, added sugars, and saturated fats

For example, you can consider the amount of sodium present in one serving of the product. Do you think a daily value of 37% contributes more or less to your diet? To understand this, you need to check the general guide to the daily value. If a product contains a 37% daily value for sodium, it indicates that this is a high-sodium product. If you consume two servings of this product, you will consume 74% of the daily sodium value. This is nearly three-fourths of the required sodium intake.

Compare Foods: You need to compare the percent daily values of food products. To do this, you need to ensure the serving size or quantity of the products is the same. You should choose products with a higher daily value for nutrients you need to consume and less of those you want to avoid.

Understand the Content Claims: You can use the percent daily value to differentiate between products, especially those that say "reduced," "low," or "light." The only thing you need to do is compare the percent daily values in every food product and see which one is lower or higher in a nutrient. You do not have to memorize or understand the definitions.

Dietary Trade-Offs: If you want to make changes to your diet by trading off some foods with others you want to eat during the day, use the dietary value percentages. You no longer have to get rid of your favorite food only because you want to lead a healthy lifestyle. When any food you prefer to eat is rich in saturated fat, you can balance it with food lower in saturated foods in other meals. You also need to watch the amount of food you eat throughout the day. This will help you control your intake of unhealthy nutrients and ensure you limit your intake to less than 100% of the daily value.

Relationship Between Daily Values and Percentages

Every nutrient you consume has a daily percentage value, and you need to meet these requirements to ensure your body receives the required nutrition. It is also important for you to understand whether you need to eat more or less of the daily value. For example, the daily value of sodium is 2300 milligrams, and this is 100%DV. As sodium isn't good for your health, you need to consume less than the actual value. We will understand this term better shortly.

Another example is dietary fiber. The daily value is 28 grams, and you need to consume more of this. The number is only the lower limit of what you need to eat. It is best to learn more about the daily value of different nutrients, so you know whether you are following a healthy diet or not.

Upper Limit

If you look at the FDA recommended value for various nutrients, you will note that the upper limit is marked as "less than." You need to limit your intake to less than the daily value listed in the table. For example, the daily intake of saturated fat is set at a limit of 20 grams. This is the 100% daily value of the nutrient you need to consume daily. The dietary guidance or advice's objective is for you to consume fewer than 20 grams of saturated fats.

Lower Limit

Similarly, the lower limit is marked as "at least" in the FDA table. For example, dietary fiber's daily value is 28 grams, and this is the 100% daily value. It indicates you need to consume at least this much dietary fiber every day.

Nutrients with no Percent Daily Value

The nutrients that do not have a percent daily value are trans fats, total sugars, and protein. Both total sugars and trans fats do not list a percent daily value on the nutrition label, but some products do list a percent daily value for proteins.

Trans Fats: The FDA and experts cannot provide a reference value that can be used to calculate the percent daily value of trans fats in foods. Therefore, it is difficult to establish this value. The Dietary Guidelines for Americans state that excess consumption of trans fats directly impacts levels of low-density lipoprotein or LDL cholesterol in your blood. This type of cholesterol, also known as bad cholesterol, increases the risk of various heart diseases. It is important to note that most manufacturers have stopped using artificial trans fats in preparing different foods since 2018.

Protein: If a manufacturer claims that the product is high in protein, then they need to list the percent daily value of protein present in the product. If the food is for children below 4 years of age or infants, the daily percentage value must be listed on the label. Otherwise, there is no need to list the daily percentage value of protein on the label.

Total Sugars: The FDA has not identified a daily value for total sugars. Thus, manufacturers cannot recommend the daily percentage value for sugars you can eat. Bear in mind that the list of total sugars in the food also includes those sugars that naturally occur in the food, along with added sugars.

Variations in Nutrition Facts Labels

Most nutrition labels use the same format as what we have discussed so far. Some manufacturers choose to label the nutrients in a different format, and the regulatory bodies authorize these formats. In this section, we will look at alternate formats – the single-ingredient sugar label and dual-column label. There are other formats manufacturers can use, in addition to the two we are reviewing in this section.

Dual-Column Labels

You can eat some products, like chips, cookies, pretzels, and biscuits, in one sitting. These products are larger than a single serving. For such products, manufacturers need to use dual-column labels that indicate the number of nutrients and calories per serving, either per unit or per package. This form of labeling aims to help people look at the number of nutrients and calories they consume when they drink or eat an entire unit or package at a time. For instance, one bag of pretzels may have a label that shows it has three servings of nutrients per container. The label will show you how many nutrients and calories would be in one package or one serving.

Labels for Single-Ingredient Sugar

Containers and packages of different foods, such as pure maple syrup, pure honey, or pure sugar, do not have to declare the quantity of added or extra sugars in grams per serving in the product. However, these containers and packages will still need to include the declaration of added sugars and the required daily value in numbers or percentages.

Regulators advise manufacturers to add the percent daily value of added sugars to the total sugar value. They need to use the "†" symbol following the added sugars' percent daily value to indicate the inclusion. They will need to add a footnote at the bottom of the label to explain the quantity of added sugars per serving. This note should also include information about the contribution of the added sugars to your daily intake.

Single-ingredient syrups and sugars are labeled in this manner to ensure consumers know that extra sugars have not been added to the product. This ensures the consumers have all the information they need about how much sugar they consume per serving.

Tips in Reading Nutritional Labels

The following are some tips to bear in mind when you read labels. Using these tips, you can stop purchasing unhealthy products. You can also watch your weight and take care of your heart.

Do Not Trust the Claims on the Box

Most people, unfortunately, trust the claims made on boxes, but it is important to remember that these are only advertisements and marketing pitches. If you find the words "light" or "low-fat," you need to remember these do not tell you the full story.

Most of these products are high in sugar, fats, calories, and salt. For example, "light" ice cream will have at least 5 grams of fat per serving. This goes to show that regular and light ice cream varieties are not very different calorically.

It is also important to stop evaluating products based on one item alone. You need to look collectively at cholesterol, fat, carbohydrate, salt, and sugar contents. As most companies want to cash in on the nutrition or diet craze, they promote their products based only on one of the items on the ingredients list and not all the other unhealthy ingredients. A product needs to pass various criteria for it to be healthy.

Read the Ingredient List and Nutrition Facts Label

Nutrition facts and ingredient lists contain the information you need to determine whether the food is healthy or not. For example, you may see the words "Trans Fat-Free" on a package of crackers, but if you read the ingredient list, it shows fats on the list. These fats include coconut oil and palm oil. These oils clog arteries like other trans fats do.

Check the Size of the Serving

The government has standardized the calculation of servings for every product many years ago, but most manufacturers still do not accurately label the serving size for their products. For instance, one serving of oil spray is quantified as 0.25 grams, which is 120th of an ounce. This is far less than a person can spray on his or her pan, even when he or she squirts the spray only once.

Read the Number of Servings per Package

A few years ago, most manufacturers labeled their products based on a single serving. One bottle of cola was only one serving. A small candy bar was also one serving. Most products have now been labeled correctly, and they contain multiple servings.

A bottle of cola amounts to 2.5 servings, and each serving is capped at 110 calories. Who in their right mind would want to drink one serving of this bottle? It is no longer a surprise why some of us are super-sized, is it?

Check the Number of Calories per Serving

Have you read the term 110 calories in a can or bottle of cola? This does not mean you drink 110 calories only. You need to multiply the number of calories per serving. As one bottle of cola comes to 2.5 servings, you consume 275 calories, and this is something you definitely need to avoid.

You should not get comfortable with the zeros either. Some manufacturers do use very small serving sizes. The FDA also states that manufacturers need to round the values down to zero, and it is for this reason that some manufacturers advertise food as fat-free or calorie-free, although they are not. If you eat multiple servings of these products, you may eat more than your required caloric intake.

Check your Caloric Intake through Fats

Yes, you will find the details of the calories you consume on the nutrition label. It is unfortunate that this number does not tell you the number of calories you consume from fat. This is the only way for you to know how to limit your fat intake. To calculate this value, you need to do a little math. Let us assume one serving of the product provides 150 calories, and 50 of these calories are from fat. This means you consume 33% of calories from fat when you eat one serving of the product.

If you do not understand how to do this, you can calculate the intake using grams. You can use this rule to calculate your intake: If the product has 2 grams or less of fat per 100 calories consumed, you can consume this product. This indicates that the fat present in the product should be 20% or less of the calories it provides.

Do not trust products that state that they only use 2% fat milk or are 99% fat-free. These labels are only based on the percentage of a serving or weight and not your caloric intake. For instance, a can of 99% fat-free soup may have more than 65% of its calories coming from fats. From research conducted by various health departments, it was found that 2% milk actually provides 35% calories in the form of fats, while 1% milk provides around 23% calories from fat.

Look at the Sodium Content

You should not worry about your daily intake of sodium. Do not worry about the daily intake or requirement since this does not matter. These values are based on government numbers and may not be helpful when it comes to your own situation. You should look at the milligrams you consume when you purchase a product.

It is important to limit your sodium intake from the number of calories you consume in every serving. The goal should be to consume only 1,500 milligrams of sodium a day. This is the Centers for Disease Control and Prevention and the American Heart Association's daily recommended intake.

Understand the Type of Fat

You need to ensure there are no partially hydrogenated fats, tropical oils, or saturated fats in the list. This means there should be no butter, lard, cocoa butter, coconut, shortening, palm oils, chocolate, margarine, part-skim, and whole dairy products. These products will damage your heart and arteries.

Monounsaturated fats, such as canola oil and olive oil, and polyunsaturated fats, such as sesame oil, soybean oil, corn oil, and safflower oil, are not as harmful as other fats, so these are acceptable. Limit your intake to ensure your caloric intake from fats is less than 20%. Otherwise, your waistline will increase, and you cannot do anything about it. It is important to remember that even good fats and oils are rich in calories.

Check the Quantity of Sugar

You need to get rid of caloric sweeteners. Look for those sweeteners and sugars that do not say "sugar," but are, in fact, sugar. Some of these products include maple syrup, corn syrup, rice syrup, honey, molasses, barley malt, malted barley, and products that end in "-ose," such as fructose and dextrose, and products which end with "-ol," such as maltitol and sorbitol.

You need to limit your intake of these sugars, especially if they are concentrated, refined, or added sugars. It is best to consume less than 5% of your total caloric intake. This means you need to restrict your intake to less than two tablespoons a day. You do not have to worry about naturally occurring sugars as these are present in fruit, vegetables, and some dairy products. Both naturally occurring and added sugars are grouped together as "sugar" in the food label.

The safest bet is to look at the ingredient list on the label, and avoid foods that have refined caloric sweeteners, especially if they are listed among the first five ingredients. I am saying this because the ingredients on a food label are listed in descending order of weight. If you find a product with sugar at the bottom of the label, then this is a better product for you to purchase.

Consume Whole Grains Only

You need to ensure that any grain you eat is a whole grain, such as quinoa, brown rice, and whole-wheat flour. Many pasta and bread products claim to be whole wheat, but if you look at the ingredients list, you will see wheat flour. This does sound extremely healthy, doesn't it? It is important to understand that this is only a refined flour. If you read further, you will see it either includes bran or whole-wheat flour. Look for products that come from whole grains only. If you pick up such a packet, you should ensure there are at least 3 grams of fiber per serving. This number indicates that the food contains whole grains.

If you think the ingredients sound too good to be true, then this is probably true. New products are launched every few months, and many of these products are developed only to cater to the latest diet. Some of these products may not even be regulated or certified by the authorities.

The FDA in Florida has recently evaluated and tested 67 diet products, and they noted all these products were labeled incorrectly. Some of these products did contain sugar, although the labels stated that they did not. Recently, consumer laboratories tested 30 low-carb bars, and they noted at least 65% of these products were labeled incorrectly. Most of these bars had salt, carbs, and sugar in them.

You should spend some extra time reading and understanding the labels on the products you want to purchase. When you continue to do this often, you will improve your understanding. You can identify the different products you enjoy and those that meet health guidelines. This will make shopping extremely easy. Your health and lifestyle are definitely worth it.

Foods to Avoid

It is difficult for people to decipher the ingredients in a food label, especially without any information about nutrition. This chapter has looked at different ways to understand a food label and the tips you can use to read nutritional labels. You need to understand the labels so you eat the right food.

Most people learn more about the fats and calories present in food through the nutrition label, but they need to focus on the ingredients present in the food. Calories are not the only important thing to look at when you reading a nutrition label. It is important to check whether the food is composed of healthy and good ingredients. For instance, if you want to follow a high-calorie diet, you need to avoid food that is made of dense ingredients. Sadly, people will purchase low-calorie food even though they cannot pronounce the ingredients on the list.

Americans eat a diet rich in processed food, which are filled with artificial flavorings, artificial additives, colorings, salts, sweeteners, preservatives, and chemicals. These ingredients are used to make sure food last longer long and taste better. These ingredients are used to ensure frozen dinners taste good, but they are going to affect your health adversely. Aside from these ingredients being harmful to you, many of the nutrients you need are stripped from the food. This makes the dish extremely unhealthy.

Look at your pantry, and go through each product. You need to check the ingredients at the back of the packaging. The following are some ingredients you need to watch out for and avoid:

Partially Hydrogenated Oil

Trans fat or partially hydrogenated oil is the fat you need to avoid. When you speak with a dietician, he or she will tell you about the fats you need to avoid, especially saturated and trans fats. These are the most harmful fats. The latter is the worst kind of fat for your heart and waistline. These fats increase the levels of LDL or bad cholesterol in your body and decrease good cholesterol levels. This is definitely not good for your health.

Foods that contain partially hydrogenated oils include donuts, popcorn, cookies, chips, cakes, and all types of fast food. When you check the ingredients list, you need to look for these words: hydrogenated, partially hydrogenated, and fractioned.

Sodium Nitrite

This ingredient is used as a preservative to increase the shelf life of various products, especially those with meat. This chemical is used to ensure fish and meat products are not contaminated with bacteria. It is also used as a salt preservative, and it can lead to dehydration. It sucks the moisture out of the product. Bacteria cannot grow in a dehydrated place, so it is the best way to prevent food from spoiling.

You can find sodium nitrite in various processed meats, such as sausages, hotdogs, bacon, packaged deli meats like ham and salami, and SPAM. When you shop for meat, stick to fresh meat from the butcher as these meats do not have this chemical.

Aspartame

This is a common artificial sweetener used in various food products, and it is made of three chemicals:

1. Methanol

2. Aspartic acid

3. Phenylalanine

These chemicals together make an additive that is sweeter than naturally occurring sugar. Most sweeteners people use, such as Splenda and Equal, have this harmful chemical. It contains zero calories. Diet Snapple, diet iced tea, diet soda, and any other food with the term "diet" has aspartame. This is the only way the food will have some flavor.

Aspartame is related to various adverse health symptoms, such as nausea, headaches, depression, irritability, and muscle spasms. People use this as a supplement as it does not contain any calories, but it can induce weight gain down the road. The long-term effects of aspartame include risk of stroke, heart disease, cancer, and diabetes. Therefore, you need to avoid anything that says "diet because chances are that the food is loaded with this ingredient.

Xanthan Gum

Xanthan gum is a sugar-like compound that is made with bacteria and fermented sugar. This does not sound good already, right? This ingredient is found in different packages and is often used to thicken food.

Have you ever wondered how a salad dressing or soup stays creamy and thick? Well, this is because of xanthan gum. This ingredient is used in sauces and salad dressings, as well as concrete and hair gel. Before you pick up a box of ice cream, look at the ingredient list, and see if it contains xanthan gum. If it does, you need to put it back.

Phosphoric Acid

How do you think soda has so many bubbles? This is because of phosphoric acid. This acid has many side effects and can lead to difficulty in breathing, dermatitis, and gastrointestinal distress. This acid can also have a negative effect on your teeth and bones because of its acidity. Phosphoric acid is also used in fertilizers, soaps, and polishes. Therefore, it is best to swap your glass of coke with water.

These are some of the harmful ingredients used in different foods, and you can find many such products in the grocery store. It is important for you to understand the food you are ingesting. Things like phosphoric acid and aspartame are claimed to be safe, but our body is not equipped to handle these chemicals. You need to eat whole, fresh ingredients without chemicals.

When you look at different foods, you need to look at the ingredients list. Even if you do not know the actual ingredients, see how many are on the list. If you see more than five ingredients on the list, chances are that this product is filled with additives and chemicals.

For example, one serving of McDonald's chicken nuggets has 38 ingredients. If you made chicken nuggets at home, how many ingredients would you use? Definitely not 38! More than half the ingredients used to make chicken nuggets in McDonald's are preservatives and flavorings. You may not eat chicken nuggets, but this holds true for various packaged products.

You can also look at how to pronounce the ingredients used to make the product. If you struggle to pronounce an ingredient or it reminds you of a chemical you read about in school, then you definitely should not eat this food. The food you eat should be filled with healthy and natural ingredients.

Chapter 7: Workouts for Paleo

To amplify the effects of just about any diet, workout is an essential ingredient. The same is applicable to the caveman diet as well.

While our ancestors never turned to any workout routine to stay fit, they had a lifestyle with zero dependence on vehicles, gym memberships, and Pilates. Instead, their daily lives involved a lot of walking, running around, cutting logs, making spears, and hunting and gathering their own food. As a result, staying fit came naturally to them. All of these awarded them with a very healthy and active lifestyle.

We are nowhere half as healthy as they used to be, despite how easily we can access gyms and various forms of workout routines. Working out for an hour and then spending the entire day glued to our couch is nowhere close to giving us a healthy lifestyle. More than working out, it is far more important to lead a lifestyle that is active. Not only do our sedentary lifestyles make us gain weight, but we also have a tendency to develop several types of chronic illnesses.

Our hectic schedules do not permit us an ample amount of time to spend on working out or just exercising generally, but reshuffling some of our priorities a bit can help us go a long way. While on a Paleo, you can follow and complete some very simple exercises, which are listed below:

Walking

This is probably the easiest and the most inexpensive form of exercise. It is perfect for just about anyone and everyone who is looking to incorporate some form of exercise or the other into their daily life.

To lose weight while following Paleo, one is required to engage in at least 30 to 45 minutes of brisk walking every day. For walking, you do not need to buy expensive clothes or shoes; you only need a pair of shoes, and you're all set. Some people prefer going barefoot while walking; this has additional benefits of its own.

Running

Much like walking, it can be done anytime and anywhere, but if you are new to it, start slowly, and let your muscles acquaint themselves to it; otherwise, you may face muscle stiffness and cramps. Start slow and increase your speed gradually. Running also works as a great stress buster and leaves you feeling energized.

Yoga

Yoga can provide your mind and body with a great amount of relaxation. It's one of the quickest and surest ways to relax and relieve yourself of stress without even stepping outside the comforts of your home.

Yoga can be practiced by just about anyone, but it is important to have some basic firsthand knowledge before beginning. Try undergoing basic training. Regular yoga practice can be beneficial in reducing your weight and toning your body.

Swimming

Another great form of exercise to instantly rejuvenate you is swimming. Unlike running or even walking, there's no repetition involved in pounding your legs.

Pilates

Although this form of exercise is relatively new, it is pretty similar to yoga. However, the primary focus here is on the strengthening of core muscles. Apart from offering you enhanced muscular endurance, it also provides better posture, balance, and flexibility. Pilates will require a bit of basic training, and you can also turn to YouTube for beginner videos, and try them at home. Be sure to practice caution to prevent any injuries.

Weight lifting

Contrary to the common misconception of weight lifting making you gain weight, it actually helps you shed stubborn fat. Helping you lose some fat and strengthening your muscles are the goals of weight lifting. However, keep in mind that weight lifting should be paired with a high-protein diet for it to show some results.

Eating Paleo already has high protein consumption as one of its musts. Lifting weights regularly also helps you stay lean and vastly improves your posture.

Elliptical Training

Elliptical training helps in loosening your muscles and also in losing weight.

Natural Movement

Your ancestors did not use elliptical trainers during the Paleolithic era. Exercise machines can fit into your time-crunched schedule, but you only work on a narrow range of muscles. These machines do not mimic the various movements you can perform outside of the gym. If you spend 30 minutes moving in the gym in a mechanical and regimented way and spend the next eight hours sitting, you are disconnecting yourself from your natural movements.

The founder of MovNat, Erwan Le Corre, calls this disconnection the human zoo syndrome. Since most people are stuck in this pattern, Corre recommends that people should learn how to move naturally. His method is broken down into 13 different skills, and these skills are categorized into manipulative (moving external objects around), locomotive (moving from one place to the next), and combative (self-defense).

You should challenge yourself and find a way to work on the different movements. You can hike, spend some time climbing a tree or even go to the local playground and swing on the monkey bars.

Strength and Conditioning

One of the most common fitness programs followed by people who are on the Paleo diet is CrossFit. This is a famous technique, and it helps you build overall fitness using different workouts. The exercises used in CrossFit use your bodyweight, and they also allow you to perform Olympic lifting. You can scale the weights to make it easier for yourself.

Arianna Brooks

Chapter 8: Celiac Disease – What Is It and Why Is It so Dangerous?

Celiac disease is an autoimmune disorder. The body of a person with an autoimmune disease has white blood cells that mistakenly attack healthy cells, thus resulting in utter chaos!

In people with celiac disease, the intestines are affected when gluten is consumed in any form. It is a genetic disorder, often running through generations in families, that affects about 1 in every 100 people in the world. In America, about two and a half million people suffer from celiac disease but remain undiagnosed. This may lead to numerous long-term complications.

As previously mentioned, gluten is a protein compound that is present in grains like barley, wheat, rye, and triticale. Thus, when a person suffering from celiac disease consumes gluten, an autoimmune reaction occurs and causes the white blood cells in the body to attack the small intestine.

As a result, the villi are damaged. The villi are small projections that resemble fingers and aid in the absorption of nutrients from food. Thus, when the villi are damaged because of the autoimmune reaction, nutrient absorption is significantly affected.

As previously mentioned, celiac disease is hereditary in nature. This means that it is passed down from one generation to another. Thus, if any of your first-degree relatives, such as a parent, sibling, or child, have the disease, you have a 1 in 10 chance of contracting it.

Arianna Brooks

Symptoms of Celiac Disease

The early signs and symptoms of celiac disease are as follows:

- Bloating of the stomach

- Pain in the stomach

- Increased gas

- Low appetite

- Diarrhea – constant or recurring

- Vomiting or instances of nausea

- Continual weight loss

- Bloody or fatty floating stools

The long-term symptoms include, but are not limited to, the following:

- Frequent and constant hair loss

- Easy bruising

- Fatigue

- Pain in the joints

- Itchy skin or dermatitis

- Delayed or missed menstrual period

Diagnoses of The Disease

If you are exhibiting the symptoms of the disease or if you feel that you may have the disease, the first step you should take is to contact your doctor or general physician. Your doctor will check your symptoms and advice that you undergo a few tests. One of the most common tests that you will be asked to undergo is a blood test.

If the blood test has a positive result for certain antibodies in your bloodstream, your doctor may advise that you undergo an upper endoscopy to determine the amount of damage that may have occurred in the small intestine.

If the endoscopy shows a considerable flattening of the villi, your doctor will advise you to adhere to a gluten-free diet or ask you to consult a registered dietician who will help you plan a gluten-free diet.

A few months after the diagnosis, your doctor may advise you to undergo another round of tests to ensure that your body is reacting appropriately to the diet.

It is advisable that all your first-degree relatives be tested for the disease because there is a high probability they might be affected, too!

Long-Term Effects on the Body

There is no specific age at which one could develop celiac disease, and the symptoms can manifest any time after the consumption of gluten-containing foods and/or medicines. If the disease is not diagnosed or if it remains untreated for a long time, it can wreak havoc in the body and sometimes even lead to long-term damage.

The long-term effects of celiac disease on the body include:

- Type 1 diabetes

- Dermatitis herpetiformis, as elaborated in an earlier chapter, is a type of skin rash that is very itchy

- Osteoporosis, a condition in which the bones become weak and very brittle

- Anemia, a condition in which there is low hemoglobin and red blood cell count in the body

- Multiple sclerosis (MS)

- Miscarriage

- Infertility

- Epilepsy

- Migraine

- Cancer of the intestines

- Short stature, especially in growing children

- Lactose intolerance

- Mineral and vitamin deficiency

- Malfunctioning of the gallbladder

- Pancreatic insufficiency

If you closely observe the long-term health effects of celiac disease, you will notice that most of the conditions arise because of the low quantity or absence of nutrients in the body. This is because of the flattening of the villi in the small intestine which further hinders the absorption of nutrients from food.

Thus, if you have even the slightest doubt that you may have celiac disease, it is better to get yourself checked by a general physician. After all, prevention is better than cure, and it is way better to be safe than sorry!

Chapter 9: Emotional Reactions

Similar to being diagnosed with any other disease or having your physical health affected in any manner, this has an impact on us mentally. Being riled by something messes with our emotions to a great extent. However, to be diagnosed with something that alters the course of your way of living completely – now that's something you need to brace yourself for, and knowing the common reactions people experience when diagnosed with celiac disease will surely help.

Anxiety

Not knowing how to deal with something so unexpected gives rise to a considerable amount of anxiety. The uncertainty of a future with all our lifestyle choices undergoing an alteration might flood our decision-making abilities – these are some very daunting thoughts for some.

Isolation

Isolating themselves has often been the first reaction many have when faced with something they desperately want to retreat from. Isolating yourself for a little while might even help to get some mental stability and peace, but any prolonged period of isolation would be deemed as unhealthy. Instead, you could reach out to those close to you and have a conversation clearly expressing how you feel, even if all you are feeling is a desperate need to run away from yourself or the gut clenching fear that the reins of your own life have been snatched away from your hands.

Insecurity and Fearing Uncertainties

It is easy to develop insecurities about yourself when thrown into an unexpected situation that shakes up your world and confidence. This is when you could look up diagnosis stories about people and their reactions to it. This helps build a secure mindset when you find relatable stories that speak to you and make you feel less alone.

Lacking Information

It's rather dangerous if you approach a situation without an ample amount of knowledge at your disposal. We fear the unknown, and the only way to remedy that is by familiarizing ourselves with all the required information that could strengthen our position in a given situation.

Depression

Depression is a treatable and common mental illness. It can change your thoughts, behavior, and mood. Depression can lead to long-lasting or continuous feelings of hopelessness, lack of interest, and sadness. These emotions and feelings can interfere with your life. Depression does run in families, and you can experience it at any point in life.

Depression is a mental disorder that is more common in women than in men. Common symptoms and signs of depression include anxiety, sadness, irritability, trouble concentrating, decreased energy, change in appetite, abnormal sleep habits, and more. This mental disorder is treated with a combination of psychotherapy and medication, but most individuals with this disorder are afraid to take treatment because of stigma and judgment. This is not a sign of weakness or a character weakness. If you know someone who is experiencing depression because of celiac disease, it is important for you to seek support and meet with a medical provider.

So, what is the connection between depression and celiac disease? Research shows that there is a link between malabsorption and brain functions. Malabsorption is your body's inability to absorb the nutrients from the food you eat. If your intestines are damaged, anything you eat will directly pass into your bloodstream, and this can increase the toxicity of your blood. These compounds can also affect your brain and its functions.

If you have celiac disease, you are at a greater risk of developing depression when compared to people without this disease. You should adopt a gluten-free diet which can alleviate the symptoms of depression if you have celiac disease. You may also be depressed after your diagnosis, because of the impact the disease has on your life. The challenges and stress that come with managing the celiac disease can lead to depression.

Arianna Brooks

Chapter 10: Treatment of Celiac Disease

At present, there is no concrete treatment available to cure celiac disease. The only way that you can address celiac disease is by adhering to a strict gluten-free diet throughout your lifetime. This means that you need to avoid all products that contain rye, wheat, barley, and triticale. These products include bread, beer, sauces, and condiments. Likewise, you should ensure that all the medication that you consume is gluten-free.

It is vital to remember that every crumb counts, and even a small crumb from the toaster or from the butter knife can be enough to cause your white blood cells to attack your small intestine, thus causing a great deal of damage. This can also give rise to a variety of symptoms – so much trouble over one single crumb.

To be specific, if you are suffering from celiac disease, once you have removed gluten from your diet, the tissues and villi of your small intestine start to heal, and all the symptoms associated with it will start to diminish.

As stated by the National Institute of Diabetes and Digestive Kidney Disease (NIDDK), *"For most people, following this (gluten-free) diet will stop symptoms, heal existing intestinal damage, and prevent further damage. Improvements begin within days of starting the diet, and the small intestine is usually completely healed—meaning the villi are intact and working—in three to six months (it may take anywhere up to two years for older adults)."*

As mentioned above, consuming any amount of gluten could result in tissue damage, whether any symptoms have manifested or not. During the initial months of being on a gluten-free diet, or until the small intestines' villi have healed, your diet may be supplemented with minerals and vitamins by your physician to replenish nutrients and remedy any deficiencies that might occur. If you have developed intolerance toward lactose, a lactose-free diet might also be required; however, this tends to return to normal within a few months of being on a gluten-free diet.

Important Aspects of Treatment for Celiac

- Strictly maintain adherence to a gluten-free diet, for a lifetime.

- Research as much as possible about the basics of how to follow a gluten-free diet and to self-manage the diet.

- Educate others in your life to comprehend the basics of a gluten-free diet.

- Adjust and acquaint yourself with the diet to let it fit into your everyday life, and make the required modifications for whatever other needs arise beyond the gluten-free aspect of the diet.

- Adjust to various potential needs, such as blood test evaluations, which include levels of minerals and vitamins.

- Evaluate the density of bone mineral with the required follow-ups, as suggested by the physician.

- Be monitored by your physician continuously to evaluate the progress that's taking place in your body, to assess your medical status, as well as to determine the changes in your condition that could call for getting additional treatment.

Living with Celiac: A Challenge

If you are suffering from it, living with celiac disease can prove to be quite the challenge, but as you start learning about it and figuring things out, managing it will become easier and even turn into your second nature. You can use the following suggestions to help ease the process of coping:

Research

Compile all the information relevant to celiac disease and also gluten-free diets. Consult your physician for additional info, and search on the Internet, but be sure to rely on websites that are reputable and that also back their claims with valid sources.

Read as much as possible, from books and health magazines to pamphlets, and buy specialized cookbooks with a central focus on gluten-free, along with books about cooking that's compatible with celiac disease specifically. Yes, such books do exist! Familiarize yourself with gluten-free groups and associations.

Knowledge is everything; it is power, a shield, a weapon – you name it! The more you know, the better you will succeed at having control over your celiac-affected life. It even eases a lot of the stress if you know when, how, and what to be watchful about.

Educate Those Around You

Educating others about something you are suffering from is just as important. From your family to your spouse, let everyone know – at least start with the basics. As specified in an earlier chapter about cross-contamination of foodstuffs, it is of utmost importance to be mindful about such risks, and avoid any scenarios that could give rise to them.

Seek Out Your Tribe

Instead of doing it alone, try to find other people who have celiac disease. There exist many local support groups, online forums, chat rooms, etc., that can support and help you through the trying times.

Professional Guidance

The beginning is always the toughest and most intimidating part of any journey. So, don't be reluctant to reach out for help from a dietician specializing in gluten-free diets, especially relative to celiac disease. A dietician can help you organize the do's and don'ts for foods you're confused about whether to eat or not.

To find a dietician in your area; you can contact the American Dietetic Association at www.eatright.org, or you could simply ask your physician to recommend one. Bear in mind that you should choose a physician and dietician who specialize in gluten-free diets and celiac disease.

Chapter 11: Autoimmune Disease – What Is It?

Autoimmune diseases are conditions where the immune system turns on your body by mistake. Normally, the immune system helps guard your body against viruses, bacteria, and other germs. When it detects invaders like these, it deploys armies of fighter cells to attack the invaders and fight them off. When the immune system is working well, it knows the difference between the proper cells and foreign ones.

With an autoimmune disease thrown into the mix, the immune system cannot tell the difference and will see a part of the body, such as the skin, the joints, or a body organ, as foreign and will produce autoantibodies, which are proteins, to attack them, even though they are healthy cells.

Some diseases target one organ only. For example, type 1 diabetes will only damage the pancreas, whereas other autoimmune diseases attack the whole body, as is the case of systemic lupus erythematosus (SLE).

So, what causes your immune system to turn on your body?

Doctors are not entirely sure why the immune system backfires on us like this, yet it is a fact that some people are more at risk of autoimmune diseases than others. Recent studies show that women are twice as likely to get an autoimmune disease than men are, and the disease will often start between the ages of 15 and 44.

Some ethnic groups are more likely to get some autoimmune diseases, such as lupus, which affects more Hispanic and African-Americans than it does Caucasians. Some autoimmune diseases, such as multiple sclerosis and lupus, tend to run in the family, but it doesn't automatically mean that every member of the family will get that disease; what they inherit is the risk of getting an autoimmune condition of some kind.

Given that the number of people with autoimmune diseases is on the rise, some researchers say that it could be down to environmental factors, such as exposure to solvents, chemicals, or infections. Further research suggests that, because we use antiseptic on everything, and children are given so many vaccinations, they don't get the exposure to germs that the previous generations did, and because of the lack of exposure, the immune system could overreact when faced with something quite harmless.

One of the biggest suspects in the rise of autoimmune diseases, however, is the Western diet. This is typically very high in sugar, fat, and processed foods, and all three are, in some way, linked to inflammation and this, in turn, can set the immune response off.

Common Autoimmune Diseases

With more than 80 autoimmune diseases detected so far, it would take forever to list them all; so here are the most common ones:

Type 1 Diabetes mellitus

The pancreas is responsible for producing a hormone called insulin, which regulates blood sugar levels. With type 1 diabetes, the immune system goes on the attack, destroying the pancreatic cells that produce insulin. This leads to high blood sugar, which, in turn, can cause damage to blood vessels, nerves, eyes, heart, kidneys, and other major organs.

Rheumatoid Arthritis

The immune system can turn on the body by producing antibodies. These attach to our joint linings, giving the green light to the immune system cells to attack those joints. This leads to inflammation, pain, and swelling, and if left untreated, the damage to the joints will eventually become permanent.

Psoriasis and Psoriatic Arthritis

Typically, our skin cells will grow, and when no longer needed, they shed. With psoriasis, the skin cells over multiply, causing a build-up of cells that turn into red, inflamed patches of skin, usually with a covering of silver-white plaque scales. Around 30% of those with the condition will go on to be affected by psoriatic arthritis, with their joints swelling painfully and going stiff.

Multiple Sclerosis (MS)

Multiple sclerosis causes damage to the coating that protects our central nervous system cells, known as the myelin sheath. When this is damaged, it affects the speed at which messages are transmitted between the spinal cord and brain and the rest of the body. This leads to numbness, balance problems, weakness, and problems with walking. There is more than one type of MS, and each type progresses differently, some faster than others, but research shows that, typically, within 15 years of the start of the disease, 50% of those with MS will need some help walking.

Systemic Lupus Erythematosus (SLE)

People who develop lupus have autoimmune antibodies attached to their body tissues. Commonly affected parts of the body include the lungs, joints, nerves, blood cells, and the kidneys.

Inflammatory Bowel Disease (IBD)

In IBD, the intestinal lining is attacked by the immune system, and this leads to rectal bleeding, diarrhea, pain in the abdomen, urgent bowel movements, weight loss, and fever. Two of the most common forms of IBD are Crohn's Disease and Ulcerative Colitis.

Addison's Disease

This disease focuses on damaging the adrenal glands, which produce androgen, aldosterone, and cortisol hormones. If there is insufficient cortisol, the body cannot use or store sugar and carbohydrates, while aldosterone deficiencies cause too much potassium in the blood and loss of sodium. Symptoms of the disease are low blood sugar, weight loss, fatigue, and weakness, among others.

Grave's Disease

With this disease, the thyroid gland, located in the neck, is under attack, making it produce an excess of its hormones. These hormones control metabolism, and an excessive amount can make your metabolism too fast, causing weight loss, intolerance to heat, a fast heartbeat, and nervousness.

One symptom that some people get is exophthalmos, commonly known as bulging eyes. Part of the Graves Ophthalmopathy, it is estimated that around 30% of those with Grave's Disease will have this, too.

Sjogren's Syndrome

Sjogren's syndrome attacks the lubricating glands around the mouth and eyes, and common symptoms are dry mouth and dry eyes, although it can also attack the skin and joints.

Hashimoto's Thyroiditis

In this condition, the immune system produces antibodies that attack the thyroid over time, causing slow destruction of the thyroid hormone-producing cells. When the levels of this hormone are too low, otherwise known as hypothyroidism, symptoms include constipation, fatigue, depression, weight gain, dry skin, and a strong sensitivity to the cold. This typically happens over months or years.

Myasthenia Gravis

This condition affects the impulses in the nerves that assist the brain in controlling muscles. When this communication is impaired, the signals cannot tell the muscles that they need to contract. The most common symptoms are muscle weakness, worsening with exercise and improving with rest. Very often, the muscles controlling facial movement, swallowing, eye movement, and opening the eyelids are affected.

Autoimmune Vasculitis

Autoimmune vasculitis is when the immune system damages the blood vessels. It can affect any or all organs, so there is a wide range of symptoms that can happen just about anywhere in your body.

Pernicious Anemia

Pernicious anemia causes deficiencies in the protein that the stomach lining cells produce. This is called the intrinsic factor and is required for vitamin B-12 in food to be absorbed by the small intestine. Deficiencies cause anemia and alterations to the body's ability has to synthesize DNA. It affects less than 1% of people in general and almost 2% of those over 60.

Celiac Disease

Those with Celiac disease are unable to consume gluten; if they consume gluten, once it gets to the small intestine, the immune system will attack and cause intestinal inflammation. Although the symptoms are similar, this is not the same as a gluten sensitivity, which is not classed as an autoimmune disease.

Guillain-Barre Syndrome

In this autoimmune disease, the nerves that mainly control the leg muscles, and occasionally, those in the upper body and arms, are attacked by the immune system. The result is weakness, occasionally very severe.

Chronic Inflammatory Demyelinating Neuropathy (CIDP)

CIDP is much like Guillain-Barre Syndrome, but, after the nerves have been attacked, the symptoms are much more prolonged. Left undiagnosed and untreated, around 30% of those with it will need to use a wheelchair.

Chapter 12: Four Reasons Why Autoimmune Diseases and Gluten Don't Mix

Not only does gluten result in a changed microbiome, leaky gut, and inflammation, it also uses a system called molecular mimicry to trigger autoimmunity directly. When a person has an autoimmune disease, he or she wants nothing more than to reverse the damage and start feeling better. Believe it or not, you can achieve both of these when you target the root cause of the disease, and in many cases, that root cause is likely to be gluten.

However, a lot of people are confused about this business of gluten, and some wonder if eliminating gluten is all that necessary, particularly those who don't have any digestive symptoms or who have tested negative for both gluten sensitivity and Celiac.

Gluten is a sneaky thing. Not everyone notices any symptoms straight away, but if they do, cutting out gluten altogether doesn't always give immediate results. However, if you do have an autoimmune disease, going gluten-free is the only way to relieve it. You see, whether you know it or not, gluten damages the body, triggering disease mechanisms and pathways, even if you have tested negative for sensitivity.

These are the four primary reasons why gluten and autoimmune diseases do not play nicely:

Gluten Triggers Inflammation

In just about every chronic disease known to man, inflammation has played a part, and that includes autoimmune diseases. In other words, those who have an autoimmune condition have likely had long-term inflammation, and this damages cells, triggering the autoimmune disease.

Environmental toxicity, lifestyle, food choices, stress, and chronic infection all play a part in inflammation and are considered to be the main triggers of the disease. If we take it a bit further, more inflammation further worsens the progression of the disease and the symptoms, making it, in effect, a vicious cycle. Whatever you do to reduce or eliminate the inflammation and kick your body's anti-inflammation mechanisms into gear will help to relieve the symptoms and, in most cases, reverse the disease progression. Studies show that one of the best ways to do this is to adopt a gluten-free lifestyle.

As an aside, we earlier mentioned food products labeled as "gluten-free" – keep in mind that these foods can also be highly inflammatory; this is down to the alternatives used in place of gluten, like potato starch and tapioca. In many cases, these alternatives cause more inflammation than gluten does.

Gluten Changes Your Gut Microbiome

The gut microbiome is made up of both good and bad bacteria that reside in the digestive tract. Research is continuing to show that this microbiome has a critical role in disease development, and some studies go as far as to suggest that autoimmune diseases could be triggered by a gut microbiome imbalance called dysbiosis.

Those who have a chronic condition or an autoimmune disease should focus on making improvements to their gut health, even if they have no symptoms that suggest something is out of kilter in the digestive system. It has also been shown that the bacterial composition in the microbiome can change incredibly rapidly – in many cases, within an hour or two of eating.

The bottom line is this – when you persist with eating foods that are known to improve the good gut bacteria, the microbiome changes for the better. Gluten has a negative influence on the microbiome and a direct effect on how autoimmune diseases develop and progress. If, for nothing else, that is a great reason to eliminate the gluten right away.

Gluten certainly isn't the only factor that affects gut microbes – medication, stress, other foods, and infections all play their part in determining which bacteria flourish in the digestive tract and which don't. However, gluten has a negative impact, altering the microbiome and influencing the autoimmune disease development and progression.

Gluten Triggers a Leaky Gut

Gluten has a significant role in the creation of a leaky gut. This happens when your digestive tract lining is damaged and cannot work properly; "holes" that should not be there appear in the lining.

With a leaky gut, particles that really should not be in your bloodstream get through the intestinal lining and start circulating through your body. Your immune system launches an attack against those particles, and the result is an inflammatory response. There is a strong belief among medical professionals that this is one of the primary mechanisms for the development of an autoimmune disease.

There is also research showing that gluten can trigger a molecule called zonulin to be released; this molecule targets the junctions that hold the intestinal lining together and breaks them down. As such, gluten is directly responsible for leaky gut, which allows the trigger into the bloodstream, resulting in the development of an autoimmune disease. Eliminate gluten from your diet, and your body can begin to heal.

Molecular Mimicry

All this means is that one molecule mimics another, a key trigger for autoimmune diseases. It works this way: A foreign invader, such as bacteria, virus, or a food particle, has a molecular structure similar to part of the human body, such as thyroid tissue. When that invader enters your bloodstream, sometimes through a leaky gut, antibodies are created, and the immune system is told to destroy the invader. The problem is that the invader is similar in structure to body tissue, so confusion reigns supreme. The body might then create more antibodies against the body tissue, and this leads to a high risk of autoimmune disease. This interaction is the most critical reason why autoimmunity and gluten simply do not mix.

Studies show that, when antibodies are created to gliadin, which is a gluten protein, they react with multiple body tissues. This is called "food immune reactivity" and is seen in cases where antibodies react with the brain, thyroid, joints, and nervous system tissues.

In layman's terms, if you have gluten sensitivity, your body makes antibodies to gliadin and other bits of the gluten molecule. These antibodies may also attach to the tissues in other parts of your body and flag them as requiring destruction.

Ditch the gluten, and these antibodies no longer get created, reducing the risk of the response.

Chapter 13: Maintaining a Gluten-Free Lifestyle while Eating Out, Traveling, and during the Holidays

While following a gluten-free diet, going out for meals might lead to anxiety. A few restaurants have "gluten-free" meals or even complete "gluten-free" menus. However, you may have concerns regarding cross-contamination and the ingredients they use to prepare these meals at the back of your mind.

Even holidays may be a source of stress because not everyone may grasp how cross-contamination happens or even how one wrong ingredient can have a big impact on the end product. Sometimes, relatives may not even take your gluten-free request seriously.

In such circumstances, how do you ensure you stay on the gluten-free track? Read on to learn some tips and tricks you can use to stay stress-free while out or during the holidays.

Tips for Dining Away from Home

Be it while traveling or while dining out, eating out when on the gluten-free diet has become easier than ever. Many regional and national chains have come up with gluten-free menus that efficiently cater to people following the gluten-free diet. Now, even a lot of fast-food chains have started offering a gluten-free option.

This said, it is still very much possible to run into trouble at a restaurant – especially if you are sensitive to trace amounts of gluten. Most of the time, the problem isn't about the food containing gluten – it is about the gluten that interacts with non-gluten ingredients by way of cross-contamination.

With the rise in the number of people asking for gluten-free meals, the restaurant industry has also become more aware of gluten-free issues and needs. This has resulted in a lot of restaurants rethinking and redesigning menus while keeping the needs of people in a gluten-free diet in mind. It is imperative to do your own research so that your diet stays gluten-free.

Here are some tips you can follow:

1. **Selection of Eating Establishment**

a. As much as possible, try to choose a restaurant that offers gluten-free options. This is not limited to the restaurant having a gluten-free menu. It can also include menus carrying naturally gluten-free items, such as fish, chicken, or meat that are not served with a flavored sauce or breaded during prep, or one that has menu items that can easily be modified to be gluten-free, such as salads without croutons or hamburgers without the bun.

b. Look up the menu of the restaurant online, and give them a call during non-busy hours to discuss your meal preferences. Preferably, call them a day prior or on the day of your visit. If possible, ask to speak directly with the chef. This will definitely increase the quality of your meal experience.

c. Choose an establishment that has extra time to discuss and prepare gluten-free items for you. Quick-service restaurants, restaurants with standard menus, and fast-food restaurants may not have the time to thoroughly check all the ingredients for you.

d. Usually, the chefs in fine-dining establishments are more aware of the concept of gluten-free and can help cater to your needs efficiently.

e. Beware of restaurants where there might be a language barrier, such that staff may not understand your dietary restrictions. Do not hesitate to request for a manager or the chef to communicate your needs to.

2. Dine Before or After the Rush Hour

Time your meal in such a way that you reach the restaurant before or after the busiest meal hours. By doing so, you will have more time to discuss your meal preferences, as well as have easier access to the chef. Remember that even the most understanding chef or server may not be able to be of any help during rush hours.

3. Briefly explain your dietary restrictions

Be polite and concise when you explain your dietary restrictions. Ask if they understand what a gluten-free diet entails. Whenever possible, give your servers a brief list of foods that might trigger you. Most people are aware of the gluten in wheat but may not be aware that there is gluten in grains like barley and rye and condiments like soy sauce. Ensure your server is interested and cooperative as he or she will be the one conveying your needs to the kitchen and handling your food. If you have the slightest doubt that the server is not clear on what you are asking for, do not hesitate to request to speak with the chef or the restaurant manager.

4. **Ask Detailed Questions**

Ask if you can see the chef to discuss your options in detail – after all, the chef is the only person who knows what exactly goes into each dish. Ask as many questions as you would like regarding the ingredients used and the prep involved. Be very specific as regards the questions you ask about each item.

Do not assume anything is gluten-free unless it's expressly mentioned to be so. Green tea might contain barley. Baked potatoes might contain a coating of flour to make the skins crispier. Egg omelets may have pancake batter in them to make them fluffier. It is best to choose dishes that do not have a sauce or a coating or dishes that can be made without a sauce.

Here is a list of popular common "gluten-free" food items and the problems associated with them:

Salads

There can be possible contamination on the chopping board used to chop up the ingredients or the addition of salad dressings that contain unsafe ingredients croutons. Request your salad to be free of any croutons or bread products, and ask for the salad to be served with the dressing on the side.

Marinades and Salad Dressings

Marinades and salad dressing might contain unsafe ingredients, such as thickeners. As much as possible, order salads with oil and a lemon wedge on the side or with oil and balsamic vinegar on the side. To be on the safer side, you could even carry a small container of salad dressing from home to avoid risking it.

Sauces and Soups

Usually, restaurants use soup bases as a foundation for a variety of sauces and soups. These bases usually contain ingredients similar to that of a broth or a bouillon – natural flavors, hydrolyzed vegetable proteins, and so on. Make sure you carefully check the ingredients before ordering. Usually, a roux (a combination of flour and butter) is used to thicken most sauces, and it is safe if you avoid its consumption. Some restaurants also use canned sauces, and you may be able to check the ingredient list.

Prime Rib and Other Meats

Sometimes, when a prime rib is prepared too rare for a customer's taste, the chef may place it in a pot of au jus until the meat is cooked to the desired doneness. This au jus may directly come from a can or a can mix and could possibly contain hydrolyzed wheat protein. While preparing most meat, chefs often use seasonings. You should verify the ingredients of any seasoning before you order. Imitation bacon bits and self-basting turkeys may also contain hydrolyzed wheat protein, so the ingredients should be verified.

Fried Foods

The oil used in restaurants may be used to fry breaded and non-breaded items, both leading to cross-contamination. In larger restaurants where French fries are fried separately in specific fryers, the risk of cross-contamination is lower.

Hash Browns, Rice, and Other Starches

A lot of pre-packaged and frozen hash browns contain added starch. Make sure you ask what other ingredients are added to starches during cooking. A lot of rice pilafs may have added ingredients or seasonings that you may have to avoid. Ordering plain steamed rice or baked rice that is cooked in water is a good choice for a gluten-free item.

Dairy Products

Often, restaurants use non-dairy products in place of dairy products to cut costs. The three most frequently used non-dairy items are non-dairy creamer, non-dairy whipped topping, and non-dairy "sour cream" topping. Make sure that all the ingredients in these non-dairy food items align with your diet restrictions.

5. Ask if They Can Further Reduce the Risk of Cross-Contamination

Request that your food be prepared using clean utensils and on a clean cooking surface. If time doesn't permit wiping down, suggest that they use foil for cooking your food so that the risk of cross-contamination is nil.

6. Be Ready to Eat an Item That Would Not be Your First Choice

Despite being informed and prepared, a restaurant may sometimes not have a satisfying gluten-free meal option for you. This can be addressed using two strategies:

a. By "pre-eating" a meal before you head out so that your hunger is in control, and there is less temptation for you to make an unhealthy eating choice.

b. By carrying gluten-free snacks, such as crackers or bread, with you. You can even carry uncooked pasta and ask the chef to prepare it for you in a clean pot.

7. Confirm Your Order Before You Start Eating

Yes, you might come across as cautious, but better safe than sorry. Confirm that your instructions were followed.

8. Thank the Staff for Their Support

Show the staff your appreciation by leaving a generous tip. If the establishment followed your instructions and provided you with a good experience, leave them a nice review on Yelp or the like. Visit the establishment again to show your support.

Sample Questions to Ask While Dining Out

Here is a list of all possible questions you can and should ask before zeroing in on an establishment to patronize or before zeroing on a dish to consume:

- Do you have a gluten-free menu?

- Which menu can items be made gluten-free?

- Do you understand what gluten is?

- Are there any crispy noodles, wontons, or croutons in the salad?

- Does your salad dressing contain any kind of flour in it?

- Does the soup contain barley or wheat flour in it?

- Is the food marinated in any sauce? Does the marinating sauce contain any teriyaki or soy sauce?

- Before being sautéed or fried, was the food coated in any kind of flour?

- Are the French fries dusted with flour? Is the oil used for French fries the same as the one used to fry breaded items?

- Do the salads or potato skins contain any meat substitutes, such as artificial bacon bits?

- Are your mashed potatoes made using real potatoes, or are they made from a pre-mix?

- Do you use any kind of imitation seafood, such as imitation crabmeat?

- Does my chosen dish come with bread?

- Will my dish be garnished with fried onions?

- Will there be a cookie with my ice cream?

- Is there a separate space to prep gluten-free food, or do you clean down space before prepping?

- Do you use separate utensils or cookware to prepare gluten-free food, or do you simply wash them before use?

- Is the grill cleaned before preparing gluten-free food?

- Do you have a dedicated fryer for gluten-free food, or do you change the oil before preparing gluten-free food?

Holidays and other Social Eating

Dining during the holiday season and on other special occasions can result in a lot of stress for people following the gluten-free diet. There's always the worry of non-availability of gluten-free items, fear of cross-contamination, and of course, the threat of being tempted by non-gluten-free items. Here is a list of easy tips and tricks that will help you enjoy a stress-free holiday season:

Get Creative

Do not let your gluten-free restrictions inhibit you from enjoying your meals. There are various gluten-free recipes available online (a bunch in this book, too) that provide you with alternatives for all your favorite holiday treats, including flour-free cakes, stuffing, cookies, bread, and pies. Get creative, look for substitutes for all your holiday baking needs, and don't be afraid to experiment with new ingredients and methods. Also, there are a bunch of pre-mixes and premade products available in the market. Check out your local health food stores and even grocery stores for the same.

Be Prepared

If you are going to be dining at someone else's house for a holiday celebration or a get-together and are not sure of the menu, carry your own food. Carry a dish or two so that you don't go hungry. If you are also unsure of the beverage options, carry a bottle or two for yourself.

Research about the Place You are Eating At

When eating at a restaurant for a meal, call ahead or look up their menu online to check if they have appropriate food choices. You can't assume they will have gluten-free options; not all restaurants are the same. If a restaurant has nothing you can eat, consider suggesting an option of a restaurant that does cater to your needs. If you will be attending a catered event, such as a wedding, call the host ahead of time and see if you can request a gluten-free option or a gluten-free meal.

Be Very Assertive

Depending upon your level of sensitivity, you may want to inform your host or your server of how severely you may react to any amount of gluten. Letting them know can help reduce your stress. Do not be afraid to ask questions, and you can even send back food if you have the slightest doubt regarding the ingredients of the dish.

Be Courteous

Do not expect everyone you may come in contact with to know what a gluten-free diet entails just because you are following this diet. Your party host or your server may not be familiar with the term. Be kind when you are required to explain your needs. If you are accidentally served something with gluten, be courteous while explaining why you can't eat it.

Stay Alert

There are many hidden sources of gluten, such as gravies, spices, sauces, and drinks. Be alert, and question everything. If you have the slightest doubt, it is better to go without the item rather than risk it.

Chapter 14: Helping Your Child Manage a Gluten-Free Diet

Your child might need to follow a gluten-free diet if diagnosed with non-celiac gluten sensitivity or celiac disease. Before cutting gluten completely out of your child's diet, it is advisable that you consult your doctor.

A gluten-free diet excludes all food items that contain wheat, rye, barley, and products derived from them, such as brewer's yeast and malt. While being gluten-free, you can still enjoy a very healthy diet full of vegetables, fruits, fish, meat, poultry, legumes, beans, and most dairy products. Following a gluten-free diet is the only way children suffering from celiac disease or non-celiac gluten sensitivity can stay healthy. There is no shot or medicine that you can take to make the disease go away.

By following the gluten-free diet, kids who suffer from celiac disease are able to efficiently absorb the vitamins and minerals from the food they consume. These vitamins and minerals are highly necessary for adequate growth. Lots of kids who follow the gluten-free diet report that they feel stronger and more energized after following the diet.

Having a child diagnosed with celiac disease is not the end of the world. There are many foods that are delicious and gluten-free, too. Fresh fruits and vegetables are gluten-free, and so are most animal proteins, such as fish and chicken. These days, there are loads of gluten-free options for items popular among kids, such as gluten-free bread, gluten-free cereal, gluten-free pizza crusts, gluten-free pancakes, gluten-free chicken nuggets, and even gluten-free ice cream! Just ensure that you carefully read the gluten-free label on the packaging before offering.

Additionally, many starches, flour, and even grain alternatives are gluten-free and can be offered to children following a gluten-free diet.

Here is a list of gluten-free flour alternatives and grains:

- Amaranth

- Buckwheat

- Rice – white, brown, and wild

- Almond meal flour

- Corn

- Coconut flour

- Cornstarch

- Millet

- Guar gum

- Pea flour

- Potatoes

- Potato flour

- Quinoa

- Soy flour

- Sorghum

- Teff

Do note that most grains are considered to be at high risk for cross-contamination. This is because, more often than not, grains are grown, milled, and processed along with gluten-containing grains. Cross-contamination occurs when gluten-free food comes into contact with gluten-containing food. Usually, this is a very small quantity, but even this small quantity can cause issues. When even a tiny amount of gluten is consumed, it can damage the small intestine and prevent nutrients from getting absorbed into the bloodstream. Whenever possible, prioritize purchasing naturally gluten-free grains, starches, and flours that have a gluten-free label on them and are certified to be gluten-free by a third-party authority.

Gluten-Free Eating for Children Over the Years

When a child is diagnosed with celiac disease or non-celiac gluten intolerance, going gluten-free is not a temporary thing – it is a commitment for life. Each stage of childhood comes with its own set of challenges. Here is how to maintain a gluten-free diet for your child during the various stages of life:

Infancy

Breastfeeding: As a mother who has been diagnosed with celiac disease, you should maintain your gluten-free diet while you are breastfeeding your child.

Formula feeding: If your child has been diagnosed with celiac disease and you are feeding the child formula, check the formula label to ensure that it is gluten-free before you start feeding your child.

Toddlerhood

When following a gluten-free diet for your child, it is imperative that you discuss it with your child's pediatrician and a pediatric nutritionist who specializes in the gluten-free diet. Always check the labels of packaged food before offering them to your child. When in doubt regarding certain ingredients, it is better to give the food a miss rather than suffer from the consequences later. Here is a list of 10 gluten-free snacks that you can offer your toddler:

1. Soft and mushy vegetables and fruits, such as avocados, kiwi, potatoes, bananas, pears, sweet potatoes, and so on. Lightly hand mash them with a fork or chop them into tiny pieces before offering them to your little one.

2. Applesauce

3. Gluten-free mac and cheese

4. Gluten-free muffins, such as zucchini muffins, pumpkin muffins, corn muffins, and banana muffins, among others

5. Cucumber sticks

6. Cream of rice – ensure that the rice is labeled "gluten-free" to rule out cross-contamination

7. Eggs – boiled, omelet, or scrambled

8. Gluten-free pancakes, such as banana almond flour pancakes, kiwi amaranth pancakes, and so on

9. Hummus with veggie sticks, such as carrot sticks, beetroot (boiled) sticks, cucumber sticks, or gluten-free crackers

10. Gluten-free toddler pouches

Remember that, along with ensuring it is gluten-free, make sure the food you are offering doesn't pose a choking hazard, such as a spoonful of peanut butter, uncut grapes, or uncut hotdogs.

School-Aged Children

The gluten-free diet and the list of foods you can and cannot consume can be confusing for anyone at any age. It may be tempting not to provide your child with the intricate details, but it is more harmful in the long run. At this age, they want to experiment and emulate their peers. You can choose their food, you can speak with their teachers, you can discuss with their servers, and do everything and anything in your power to protect them. However, in the long run, it is their choices that make or break the diet.

Keeping things on a "need to know basis" may work now, but it won't work forever. Rather than beat around the bush, face the disease head-on by explaining your child's disease to them from the start. Take them on grocery runs, teach them how to read the labels, play toy food parties with gluten-free food items, and encourage them to help you with the garden. The only way you can help them forward is by keeping them aware.

Packing a Gluten-Free Lunch

Sometimes, many parents prefer to send packed lunches with their kids instead of letting the child eat from the school cafeteria. This can help ease a lot of concerns surrounding the ingredients used and the prep done by the cafeteria staff. Most parents report that they get stuck while packing lunches because they feel confused over what is gluten-free and not. Use the tips in the next section to keep your kid's lunches delicious, as well as gluten-free.

Lunch Packing Tips to Keep Things Gluten-free

1. Spend at least a week or two experimenting with various new products and recipes. Keep three boxes in your kitchen labeled "like it," "love it," and "hate it." Allow your child to write the name of each product or recipe on a small piece of paper and put it in the aforementioned boxes. Do not limit this experiment to just cooked food; also include raw fruits and vegetables

2. Get creative when it comes to spreads, jams, dips, condiments, and so on. Make sure you store them in an airtight container and double secure them in a plastic bag. Make sure that upon purchase, they have a gluten-free tag on them.

3. If your child is an underweight picky eater who needs to gain weight post-diagnosis, don't worry. Calorie powers, nutritional shakes, and power bars can pack a punch; just make sure the

packaging mentions "gluten-free." Consulting with a certified dietician can also help you with meal planning.

4. When you stumble across a meal that's a winner, send enough with your child to share. This will help your child's peers accept their dietary choices and help your child gain acceptance into the group.

5. Discuss with your child how trading food can be risky for their health, and while they can share their food with peers, accepting most foods in return could pose a risk to their health.

25 Gluten-Free Snack Ideas for Kids

1. Corn tortilla chips with guacamole or salsa

2. Gluten-free pretzels

3. Gluten-free baked corn dogs

4. Celery sticks smeared with peanut butter and topped with raisins (ants on a log)

5. Gluten-free toast with mashed avocados

6. Cucumbers cut into fun shapes with hummus

7. Berry yogurt parfaits

8. Gluten-free crackers topped with cheddar, bacon, and chives

9. Pumpkin bars with a brownie bottom

10. Fruit popsicles

11. Kale muffins

12. Kale chips

13. Gluten-free tortillas with cheese and veggies (Gluten-free quesadillas)

14. Apples with peanut butter

15. Popcorn

16. Rice cakes

17. Gluten-free crackers with cheese

18. Applesauce

19. Frozen grapes

20. Fruit salad

21. Potato chips and gluten-free dip

22. Candy corn mini muffins

23. Gluten-free crackers topped with mashed bananas and peanut butter

24. Butternut squash pizza slices

25. Gluten-free tortillas filled with gluten-free meat, cheese, mayonnaise, and lettuce

Chapter 15: Healthy Food Substitutes to Consider

If you like the idea of improving your health and losing weight, you are not alone. You may also feel a little less enthusiastic because diets prevent you from eating what you like. More than 50% of people want to lose weight, but only a few do something about it. Does this sound familiar to you? If yes, control yourself. You can swap different foods with healthier alternatives, and you can make it through the week eating only healthy foods. You will no longer feel hungry or deprived.

These delicious and easy swaps will help you stick to your breakfast, lunch, and dinner plans. You can also find a way to switch to healthier snacks and desserts. These options are a painless way for you to save yourself a ton of calories. You can also see a difference in the scale. When you switch to these alternatives, you consume more nutrients every time. In this chapter, we will look at the different alternatives or substitutes.

Eat Whole Eggs instead of Egg Whites

Do you know whether you should eat the egg yolk or not? This is an important question and one that everybody asks. Eating whole eggs is a healthier option when compared to egg whites. The yolk has choline, which is a nutrient that helps your body burn fats, so you should opt for whole eggs. This is one of the easiest ways for you to lose weight.

Avoid Flavored Oatmeal

It is best to replace flavored oatmeal with unsweetened oatmeal. There are some exceptions to this rule, but flavored oatmeal is a calorie and chemical landmine. It is stripped of all nutrients. If you want to reduce your additives and sugar intake, eat a bowl of rolled oats with water. Add some cinnamon, honey, and nuts for some flavor. If you are the type of person who may forget about it, you can leave a bowl of oats in the microwave.

Eat Nuts instead of Granola

Granola is an innocent topper. You can add this to yogurt, but it is full of sugar. If you want an extra crunch with your meal without adding extra sugar or calories, top the yogurt off with some nuts and seeds. If you want to add some sweetness, you can add some honey or maple syrup.

Eat Avocado instead of Jam

Most people choose to begin their day with jam-topped toast. You may miss out on an opportunity to eat something healthy and filling. Increase your nutrient intake by adding more fruit and vegetables to your meal. Avoid eating a fruit spread. You can also mash an avocado and add that to the top of your toast. Drizzle some lemon juice on the avocado, and top it off with some vegetables. The fats from the avocado are monounsaturated or healthy fats. It also contains fiber, and this will keep you satisfied and full until the afternoon. This is especially true when you pair this sandwich with an egg.

Eat Vegetables instead of Cheese

When you begin your day with an omelet or egg sandwich, it is important for you to swap the cheese with vegetables. This is a great way for you to reduce your intake of calories, sodium, and fat. Onion, spinach, and tomato are good options for sandwiches, but any combination will taste good with eggs. If you want to reduce your time in front of the stove, chop the vegetables before time. The only thing you need to do is to toss them on the pan in the morning. This will save you time and also ensure you eat healthily.

Replace Organic Whole Milk with Creamer

A traditional creamer is made using a combination of soybean oil, corn syrup, water, and sugar. These creamers also have a stabilizer called carrageenan, which is associated with inflammation. This is going to keep getting worse. One serving of this creamer is one tablespoon, while an unmeasured or average pour of this creamer is equal to four tablespoons. One tablespoon of this dish amounts to 35 calories, with 6 grams of sugar and 1.5 grams of fat. So, when you pour the creamer into your dish, you need to multiply this by four times. If you add another cup of this creamer, your intake is going to go up. The best thing to do would be to use natural creamer. Alternatively, you can use organic whole milk and add a little cinnamon to give it some flavor. The calcium in the milk is a great way to counter the effects of caffeine. This is also a great way to add vitamins A, B12, and D, which are all important for your health. You need to be careful about what you are adding to your coffee.

Arianna Brooks

Eat English Muffins and not Bagels

You should do your best to avoid the neighborhood deli. There is nothing good about the food in this deli. If you look at the nutritional statistics, one bagel is equivalent to four slices of white bread, and both are unhealthy for you. This morning staple is rich in calories but also does not have any nutrients, such as protein or fiber. This means you will not be energized throughout the day. The healthier option is to eat whole-grain English muffins. These have starchy goodness and only have half the calories that a bagel has. It also has 4 grams of filling protein and 3 grams of fiber.

Eat Bacon instead of Sausage

While bacon is a better option, it is important to note that sausages are healthier than bacon. However, as bacon is easy to eat in moderation, it is a healthier alternative. You can cut it thin so it absorbs less oil when compared to sausages. Therefore, it is best to eat bacon instead of a sausage as it only has 3 grams of fat and 43 calories.

Drink a Bloody Mary instead of a Mimosa

Mimosas are made with a lot of sugar and are thus higher in calories. A Bloody Mary is lower in calories and comes with add-ons, such as celery. This is a better drink to have during brunch than mimosa as it has less sugar, more vitamin C, and around 125 calories. It is also rich in vitamin A and potassium from tomato juice. If you want to drink something else at the end of brunch, you can wash it down with a virgin Bloody Mary. Avoid drinking too much alcohol. The drink almost tastes the same, and you can save yourself from a hangover and any excess calories.

Eat Chili instead of Creamy Soup

You need to avoid soups that are rich and creamy. Choose cans and recipes that rely on purees, chicken broth, meat, beans, and vegetables as a base. This is an easy way to reduce your caloric intake and cut back on the fat you eat. Chili is a favorite for everybody, and it provides loads of protein and fiber. It is comforting and hearty. You can look for some amazing chili recipes in the last chapters of this book.

Eat Bowls instead of Burritos

Depending on the size of the wrap, you can eat anywhere between 250 to 470 calories. This is when you choose a flour-based wrap. If you want to get the flavor you want without eating too much, you can choose a bowl instead. Fill up the bowl with healthy vegetables, salsa, yogurt, and a little rice. This is a healthy meal.

Use a Corn Tortilla instead of a Flour Tortilla

Do you love tortillas? Can you not handle the idea of ditching a tortilla? Well, switch from a flour-based tortilla to a corn tortilla. The latter has fewer calories and more fiber when compared to the former.

Arianna Brooks

Use Hummus instead of Mayo

If you love grabbing a sandwich or find making a sandwich easier at home, ditch the mayo, and use hummus instead. One tablespoon of mayonnaise has 10 grams of fat and 95 calories. One tablespoon of chickpea-based hummus has 1.2 grams of protein, 25 calories, and 1.4 grams of fat. Plus, it adds more flavor to your sandwich than mayonnaise. This lowers your caloric intake, thereby helping you lose weight.

Eat Side Salads instead of Fries

You may grab a small serving of fries every time you eat a burger. This is only going to add another 230 calories. Instead of eating a serving of fries, eat a side salad. You can save at least 200 calories. The nutritional statistics will vary based on where you eat your food, but you can grab an entire salad instead of eating anything unhealthy. This is a smarter choice. The only thing you need to be careful about is going light on your dressing to reduce your caloric intake. If you love adding dressing, choose low-calorie options to help you lose weight.

Use Regular Salad Dressing

Vitamins K, E, D, and A are great vitamins, and they are fat-soluble. These are found in salads. Your body cannot absorb these vitamins if you do not have enough fats in your body. Having said that, you are not doing anything good for your body by using fat-free dressing. If you cannot deal with not eating a full-fat dressing, you need to look for one that is low in sugar. Most manufacturers that remove fat from any product tend to add sugar to the food for flavor. You can use any salad dressing for this, but read the ingredient list to ensure you pick the right product.

Eat Popcorn, Fruits, or Vegetables instead of Chips

Do you eat a salad or sandwich with a packet of chips? It is time to get rid of this habit. Chips do not add too much to the table when it comes to nutrition. There are more filling and healthier options, and these options also pack only a few calories. Fruits, popcorn, and baby carrots are healthier options, and these are better for you.

Use Goat Cheese instead of Low-Fat Cheese

Full-fat dairy is rich in calories, and it is filling. For this reason, some people who eat full-fat dairy products are less likely to be obese than people who prefer to eat low-fat dairy products. The latter is often filled with preservatives and additives. If you want to make the most of your caloric intake, eat feta cheese or goat cheese. These cheeses have CLA or conjugated linoleic acid, which is a form of fat that reduces the risk of cancer and heart diseases. It can also help you burn fat. If you like cheese, eat full-fat cheeses.

Prefer Homemade Chocolate Trail Mixes to Candy

Are you craving chocolate? Do not grab a bar of Snickers or any other chocolate. If you want to satisfy your cravings, you may grab a bowl of candy or sweets. You should avoid this and find a healthy substitute. If you want to eat chocolate, do not make that the hero of your dish, but make it one of the many ingredients you use. You can use different ingredients along with chocolate to increase your intake of nutrients while decreasing your caloric intake. You will still get the sweet and creamy flavor you want.

At the start of the week, mix some raw nuts and popcorn. Combine this mixture with dark chocolate chips and unsweetened dried fruit. To ensure you do not eat too much homemade trail mix, measure the servings, and store the mix in your pantry. You can also keep a bag of this in your desk drawer. Doing this will ensure you eat snacks with protein, whole grains, healthy fats, chocolate, and fiber. Eat this whenever you are extremely hungry.

Eat Kale or Jicama Chips

If you love eating chips and have a salt tooth, you will find it hard to give this up. However, given that there are so many alternatives to chips, this is not impossible. Let us put things into perspective. One pack of Lay's has 10 grams of fats, 2 grams of protein, 1 gram of fiber, and 160 calories. If you eat the same quantity of Jicama chips, you will eat 2 grams of protein, 5 grams of fiber, 1.5 grams of fat, and 100 calories. This is impressive, isn't it? Jicama and kale chips do not look like regular chips, but these are the best alternatives.

Eat Hummus with Vegetables instead of Pita Bread

Most people believe pita bread is a healthy snack, but if you look at its nutritional values, you will see it is no different from white bread. Therefore, you need to ditch the pita bread and eat hummus with fresh vegetables. The latter is lower in calories and is rich in nutrients. This will keep you healthy.

Eat Croissants instead of Muffins

Do you eat a slice of pastry and drink a cup of green tea to get through the 3 p.m. slump? Well, this is not a very good idea. Instead of choosing a muffin, eat a croissant because you can save yourself from eating 250 calories.

Eat Whole Fruits instead of Juices

Whole fruit has fewer calories and more fiber. Fiber is a nutrient that can control your weight and lower the risk of heart disease. It is healthier than fruit juice; therefore, it is best to pick a whole fruit.

Prefer Grass-Fed to Conventional Beef

When it comes to burgers or steaks, you need to choose grass-fed beef. The reason for this is that grass-fed beef has fewer calories and is leaner than conventional beef. A seven-ounce ounce conventional, lean strip steak has 16 grams of fat and 386 calories. A grass-fed, seven-ounce strip of beef only has 5 grams of fat and 234 calories. Grass-fed meat is rich in omega-3 fatty acids, which reduces the risk of cardiovascular diseases.

Eat Spaghetti Squash instead of Pasta

It is easy to drop a box of spaghetti into boiling water. Instead of doing this, you should use spaghetti squash. Bake it, and remove the strings of squash from it. This allows you to increase your intake of vegetables and reduce your caloric intake in the process. One cup of semolina spaghetti has 169 calories, whereas one cup of spaghetti squash only has 31 calories.

Avoid Sushi Rolls

A lot of people love eating sushi, but this dish is abundant in calories. When you order sashimi at a restaurant, you can reduce your caloric intake and get rid of any empty carbohydrates. Wild yellowtail tuna or wild salmon sashimi with a seaweed salad or edamame make a filling, flavorful, and well-rounded meal.

Eat Cauliflower Rice

Cauliflower is a cruciferous vegetable that is low in carbohydrates and calories. If rice is a staple, you can swap it with cauliflower rice. This cruciferous vegetable has begun to make its way into various recipes, including fried rice, pizza, and mashed potatoes. Grate a cup of cauliflower, and add it to your rice recipe. Avoid using nutrient-deficient and highly refined white rice. This will save you at least 145 calories. This is impressive, isn't it? You can use cauliflower in different ways to reduce your caloric intake.

Eat Greek Yogurt

You may love eating sour cream and top your tacos and chili with it. Avoid doing this. Use Greek yogurt instead of tacos and cilantro seasoning to add some flavor. This will save you from the fat and calories and will also add some protein to your plate. This is a win-win situation.

Eat Thin Crust Pizzas

The crust of your pizza is where the maximum number of calories lies. Pizzas are not only full of calories, but the crust does not have any nutrients. The crust is made from refined white flour, and this only increases blood sugar levels. You will crave more. You need to eat less crust, and if you love pizza, it is best to choose a thin-crust pizza over a deep dish, stuffed crust, or regular crust pizza.

Do Not Eat Too Much Ice Cream

If you love ice cream, you cannot control yourself from eating a bowl every other day. You can eat nice cream instead. Nice cream is a creamy dessert that is like ice cream but is made using bananas. You can add whatever topping you want to a bowl of nice cream. It is the best way to control your cravings when you work on losing weight.

If you want to make it, all you need to do is blend two frozen bananas and add a spoon of unsweetened cocoa powder. Blend until the mixture has a creamy consistency. It will be as soft as ice cream. Scoop this mixture into a bowl, and freeze it for a few minutes before you eat it. Half a bowl of this will only add 110 calories to your intake, whereas a half-cup of Ben and Jerry's gives you 250 calories. Do you not want to roll your sleeves up and make something? Well, find a diet ice cream.

Avoid Milk Chocolate

It is best to eat dark chocolate instead of milk chocolate because the former has flavanols, which are plant-based nutrients. Flavanols in cocoa can reduce blood pressure, fight cell damage, and improve blood flow to the heart and brain. Having said that, too much of anything, even dark chocolate, can increase weight. Therefore, you need to be careful about portion control. Do not buy a large bar of dark chocolate, but buy individually wrapped pieces to control your intake.

Use Muffin Tins instead of Cake Pans

If you love desserts, do not worry because you do not have to give them up just because you want to lose weight. The only thing you need to worry about is eating desserts in moderation. If you want to control your portions, swap your cake tin with a muffin pan. Do not make a batch of brownies in a large pan because you will dive in with your fork. You should make them in portioned muffin tins. This will make it easier for you to indulge in just one muffin. Another great thing about using muffin tins is that you can pack these muffins in a Ziplock bag and leave them in the freezer. This way, you need to do some work before you can dig one muffin out. This will be enough to stop you from eating more.

Use Cinnamon instead of Sugar

It is best to swap sugar for cinnamon to add some sweetness to a dish. You need to think about the recipe you are using and see how you can get the best flavor without removing all the tasty ingredients. One of the best ways to do this is to use spices. When you use nutmeg or cinnamon instead of sugar, you can add a lot of flavor to the dish. These spices will reduce your caloric intake and help you control your blood sugar levels.

Avoid Cookies

If you love cookies, you need to find a way to dial back on them. Try to swap your intake of refined sugar by preparing a batch of energy bites. You can eat these instead of your usual sweet treats. The best part about this is that you do not have to bake them. Look at some of the recipes later in this book to make your own sweet treats.

Applesauce instead of Sugar

If you love baking at home, you may want to use sugar to sweeten the products. If you want to lead a healthy lifestyle, you need to swap sugar for applesauce. Use the ratio 1:1 to swap sugar out with applesauce. If you do choose to use applesauce, you need to reduce the other liquids you add to the bowl. One cup of unsweetened applesauce has only 100 calories, whereas one cup of sugar has 770 calories. Depending on the serving size you make, you can save anywhere between 25 and 250 calories.

Organic Fruit Leathers instead of Gummies

One cannot deny that gummies from the store are delicious. It is important to note that these gummies are only gelatin mixed with food dye and sugar. This means they are not nutritious. When you crave fruity treats, you can make your gummies at home or buy some fruit leather, which is made from vegetables and fruit.

Chapter 16: Gluten-Free Buyer's Guide

Gluten is a group of proteins found in a few grains, such as barley, wheat, and rye. Gluten helps food retain its shape by providing the required moisture and elasticity. It also allows bread and other products to rise, giving them a chewy and soft texture.

Most people can eat gluten, but it is important to avoid food with gluten to prevent any health effects, especially if you have gluten sensitivity or celiac disease. As many foods have gluten ingredients, it is important for you to determine what ingredients are used to manufacture the product. This means you need to read the ingredients carefully and understand what the food contains.

Whole Grains

Below, you can find a list of whole grains you can consume if you are following a gluten-free diet. Some grains do contain gluten, while others are gluten-free. You need to read the labels before you purchase any product, and we have looked at the different aspects to consider when you read labels in the sixth chapter. It is important to remember that gluten-free whole grains may have some gluten in them, especially if they are processed or manufactured in the same facilities as gluten foods.

For instance, oats are processed in facilities where wheat and other gluten compounds are processed, leading to contamination. For this reason, you need to confirm whether the oats you purchase are certified free of gluten.

Gluten-Free Whole Grains

- Brown rice

- Sorghum

- Teff

- Wild rice

- Tapioca

- Quinoa

- Arrowroot

- Millet

- Buckwheat

- Amaranth

- Oats – you need to read the label and understand the ingredients used

Grains to Avoid

- Barley

- Triticale

- Wheat products, such as wheat berries, whole wheat, durum, bulgur, kamut, farro, graham, farina, bromated flour, spelt, etc.

- Rye

These grains contain gluten, and they are used to make such products as pasta, bread, crackers, baked goods, snack foods, and cereals.

Vegetables and Fruits

All fresh vegetables and fruits are gluten-free. However, some processed vegetables and fruits contain gluten because they have additives or flavoring. Gluten-containing ingredients that are added to vegetables and fruits include modified food starch, maltodextrin, and malt.

Vegetables and Fruits to Eat

The below list is not exhaustive, but it has some examples of fresh vegetables and fruits. You can enjoy these when you follow a gluten-free diet.

- Apples

- Citrus fruits, such as grapefruit, lime, and oranges

- Green beans

- Berries

- Peaches

- Pears

- Bell peppers

- Cruciferous vegetables, such as broccoli and cauliflower

- Carrots

- Bananas

- Greens, such as kale, Swiss chard, spinach, fenugreek, and Amaranthus

- Starchy vegetables, such as corn, potatoes, and squash

- Radishes

- Mushrooms

- Onions

Vegetables and Fruits to Check

Canned Vegetables and Fruits

Most canned vegetables and fruits are preserved with additives and sauces that contain gluten. If you want to eat canned vegetables and fruits, you need to pick the products canned with natural juices or water, which are gluten-free.

Frozen Vegetables and Fruits

These may contain some added flavors and sauces, both of which contain gluten. It is best to purchase plain varieties because these will be gluten-free.

Dried Vegetables and Fruits

Some dried varieties may contain gluten additives. Most unsweetened, plain, and dried vegetables and fruits are gluten-free.

Pre-Chopped Fruits and Vegetables

These foods may be contaminated with various gluten additives depending on where and how they are prepared.

Proteins

Most foods contain protein, especially plant-based and animal sources, and these sources are free of gluten. Having said that, some products, such as malt, soy sauce, and flour, are used as flavorings or fillers. These are added to rubs, marinades, and sauces, paired with various protein sources.

Gluten-Free Proteins

- Legumes, such as peas, lentils, peanuts, and beans

• Seeds and nuts

• Traditional soy foods, such as edamame, tofu, and tempeh

• Poultry, such as fresh turkey and chicken

• Seafood, such as scallops, fresh fish, shellfish

• Red meat, such as pork, bison, lamb, and beef

Proteins to Check

• Meat substitutes, such as vegetarian patties and jackfruit

• Ready-to-eat proteins, such as dinners and other frozen food

• Ground meats

• Processed meats, such pepperoni, hotdogs, sausage, bacon, and salami

• Cold cuts and lunch meats

• Proteins that have been combined with sauces or seasonings

Proteins to Avoid

• Seitan

• Avoid any poultry, fish, or meat that has been bred

- Proteins that have wheat-based soy sauce

Dairy Products

Most dairy products do not have any gluten, but they do contain additives for more flavor. Therefore, you need to check the products to see if there is any gluten in them. Some gluten-containing ingredients used in dairy products include modified food starch, thickeners, and malt.

Gluten-Free Dairy Products

- Cottage cheese

- Milk

- Cheese

- Yogurt

- Butter and ghee

- Cream

- Sour cream

Dairy Products to Check

- Flavored yogurts and milk

- Ice cream if it is mixed with additives that contain gluten

- Processed cheese products, such as spreads and sauces

Dairy Products to Avoid

- Dairy products with malt

Oils and Fats

Oils and fats are gluten-free naturally. In most cases, these oils and fats are mixed with additives that have gluten in them. This is done to thicken the oil or add some flavor to it.

Gluten-Free Oils and Fats

- Avocados and avocado oil

- Olives and olive oil

- Butter and ghee

- Coconut oil

- Seed and vegetable oils, such as canola oil, sunflower oil, and sesame oil

Fats and Oils to Check

- Oils with added spices or flavors

- Cooking sprays

Beverages

There are different types of gluten-free beverages you can enjoy if you have celiac disease. That said, some alcoholic beverages are made using gluten-based compounds. Some alcoholic beverages are made using barley, malt, and other grains that contain gluten. You need to avoid this if you want to follow a gluten-free diet.

Gluten-Free Beverages

- 100% fruit juice

- Lemonade

- Water

- Coffee

- Tea

- Some alcoholic beverages, such as beer, wine, and hard ciders if they are made from gluten-free grains, such as sorghum or buckwheat

- Energy and sports drinks

- Soda

It is important to note these beverages are all gluten-free, but it is best to consume most of these in moderation because of their alcohol and added sugar content.

Beverages to Check

- Pre-made smoothies

- Beverage made with added mix-ins or flavorings, such as coffee coolers

- Distilled liquors, such as whiskey, vodka, and gin.

These products, even when labeled as gluten-free, must be checked because they might cause some unwanted reactions

Beverages to Limit

- Beers made from gluten-containing grains

- Ales made from gluten-containing grains

- Lagers

- Non-distilled liquors

- Wine coolers and other malt beverages

Condiments, Spices, and Sauces

Most people overlook condiments, spices, and sauces, but these may contain gluten. Most condiments, spices, and sauces are gluten-free. Having said that, some gluten-containing ingredients are mixed with these condiments, spices, and sauces to enhance their flavor. They can also be used as flavor enhancers and stabilizers. Some common ingredients added to condiments, spices, and sauces are maltodextrin, wheat flour, modified food starch, and malt.

Gluten-Free Condiments, Spices, and Sauces

- Coconut aminos
- Distilled vinegar
- Apple cider vinegar
- White vinegar
- Tamari

Condiments, Spices, and Sauces to Check

- Salad dressing
- Ketchup and mustard
- Pasta sauce
- Relish and pickles
- Barbecue sauce
- Stock and bouillon cubes
- Worcestershire sauce
- Dry spices
- Salsa

- Tomato sauce

- Rice vinegar

- Marinades

- Gravy and stuffing mixes

- Mayonnaise

Condiments, Spices, and Sauces to Avoid

- Wheat-based teriyaki sauce and soy sauce

- Malt vinegar

Ingredients to Avoid or Limit

The following is a list of food additives and ingredients that have gluten in them. You need to avoid these:

- Gluten stabilizer

- Teriyaki or soy sauce

- Malt-based ingredients, such as malt extract, malt syrup, and malt vinegar

- Wheat-based ingredients, such as whole wheat flour and wheat protein

- Maltodextrin and modified food starch; the former is made from wheat, and this information will be present on the nutrition facts label

- Emulsifiers listed on the label

If a product you want to purchase does not contain gluten, you can directly speak with the manufacturer to check.

What Conditions Can You Improve Through a Gluten-Free Diet?

A gluten-free diet, as mentioned earlier, is recommended for people who have celiac disease. As we read earlier, celiac disease is a condition that triggers a response from the immune system when you eat food with gluten. If you have sensitivity towards gluten but do not have celiac disease, you can still follow a gluten-free diet. The symptoms of gluten sensitivity include stomach pain, diarrhea, and bloating.

A study conducted in 2018 by Rej A and Sanders D S suggests that a gluten-free diet is suitable for a person with irritable bowel syndrome. This disorder is characterized by different symptoms, such as gas, stomach pain, constipation, and diarrhea.

Arianna Brooks

Chapter 17: Gluten-Free Recipes for Kids

Gluten-Free Applesauce

Ingredients

- 8 apples, peeled, cored, and roughly chopped

- 1/2 cup white sugar

- 1 1/2 cups water

- 1 teaspoon ground cinnamon

Method

1. Place the apples at the bottom of a saucepan, and heat over a low flame.

2. Add in the sugar and cinnamon, and mix well.

3. Once the sugar starts melting, add in the water, and mix well.

4. Cover the saucepan and cook over a medium flame for about 20 to 30 minutes or until the apples are soft.

5. Cool to room temperature.

6. Once cooled, mash using a potato masher or a fork.

7. Serve immediately, or store in the refrigerator in an airtight container.

Greek Style Gluten-Free Scrambled Eggs

Ingredients

- 2 tablespoons butter

- 2 teaspoons water

- 6 eggs

- 1 cup crumbled feta cheese

- Salt, to taste

- Pepper, to taste

Method

1. Add the butter to a skillet, and heat over a medium-high flame.

2. In a bowl, whisk together the water and eggs until lightly frothy.

3. Pour this mix into the pan.

4. Add in the feta cheese and continue cooking, occasionally stirring to scramble the eggs.

5. Once the eggs are done, sprinkle salt and pepper to taste.

6. Serve hot with a side of gluten-free toast.

Arianna Brooks

Quick Gluten-Free Almond Flour Pancakes

Ingredients

- 2 teaspoons oil, or as needed
- 2 cups almond flour
- 4 eggs
- 1/2 cup water
- 2 tablespoons maple syrup
- 1/2 teaspoon salt

Method

1. Gently whisk water, maple syrup, and eggs together in a bowl until well combined.

2. In another bowl, gently mix together almond flour and salt.

3. Pour the wet ingredients into the dry ingredients, and whisk well until the batter is smooth.

4. Add some oil to a skillet, and heat over a medium flame.

5. Scoop the batter by the spoonful, and pour into the hot skillet.

6. Continue cooking until there are bubbles on the surface of the pancake and the edges dry out.

7. Flip the pancake over, and cook until well browned – for about 3 to 5 minutes.

8. Repeat with the remaining batter until all the pancakes are done.

9. Serve hot, topped with maple syrup and some whipped cream on the side.

Sweet or Savory Gluten-Free Cheese Waffles

Ingredients

- 1 cup mozzarella cheese, shredded

- 2 large eggs

Method

1. Before you start cooking, preheat your waffle iron.

2. Whisk the eggs in a bowl, and add in the shredded mozzarella cheese. Mix well.

3. Pour about 1/4th of the batter onto the preheated waffle iron. Spread the batter out from the center to the sides using a spoon.

4. Close the waffle iron, and cook until the waffle is well browned and the steaming stops. This should take about 3 minutes. Do not overcook as that makes the waffle very chewy.

5. Repeat with the rest of the batter until all the waffles are done.

6. Serve hot, topped with a dollop of butter and fruits or vegetables of your choice.

"Phirni" Gluten-Free Starch Pudding

Ingredients

- 1 1/3 cups cornstarch

- 12 whole cardamom seeds

- 4 cups milk

- 3/4 cup ground almonds

- 1/2 cup white sugar, or to taste

- Rosewater to taste

- 1/3 cup blanched almonds, slivered

Method

1. Add the cornstarch to 2 cups of milk, and mix well until the cornstarch is dissolved.

2. Add the remaining milk to a thick-bottomed pan, along with ground almonds and cardamom. Heat until the milk starts bubbling.

3. Reduce the flame to a medium flame, and add in the milk in which you have previously dissolved the cornstarch.

4. Add in the rosewater and sugar to taste.

5. Continue boiling the mixture for about 3 minutes while constantly stirring it.

6. Fish out the cardamom seeds from the mixture and discard.

7. Transfer the prepared mixture into serving bowls.

8. Serve hot or chill before serving.

Quick and Easy Gluten-Free Fluffy Cloud Bread

Ingredients

- 6 large eggs, separated

- 1/4 pound cream cheese, very soft

- 1/2 teaspoon cream of tartar

- 2 tablespoons white sugar

Method

1. Turn up your oven to 350 degrees F (175 degrees C), and allow it to preheat for at least 20 minutes. Use parchment paper to line a baking sheet.

2. Combine the egg whites and cream of tartar together in a large bowl, and whisk well until stiff peaks form.

3. Combine the egg yolks, sugar, and cream cheese together in a separate bowl using a small wooden spoon. Then, use a handheld eggbeater to whisk the ingredients well until they form a smooth mixture and no granules remain.

4. Gently add the egg whites to the cream cheese mixture, and fold well. Do not over mix, or else, the egg whites will deflate.

5. Scoop the mixture using an ice cream scoop to form 10 to 12 buns.

6. Place in the preheated oven, and bake for 30 minutes or until the cloud bread is lightly browned.

7. Serve topped with some peanut butter and bananas or with some jam.

Gluten-Free Green Zucchini Waffles

Ingredients

- 1 1/2 cups shredded zucchini

- 1 1/2 teaspoons vegetable oil

- 1 egg

- 1/8 teaspoon onion powder

- 1/4 cup dry potato flakes

- 1/2 pinch salt

- 1/8 teaspoon baking powder

Method

1. Following the manufacturer's instructions, preheat your waffle maker.

2. Combine the zucchini, vegetable oil, salt, egg, and onion powder together in a large mixing bowl. Add in the baking powder and potato flakes, and mix well until the batter is well combined.

3. Pour about ½ cup of the prepared batter onto the center of the preheated waffle iron. Spread the mixture out using a spoon.

4. Close the lid, and cook the waffle until the waffle is crispy and stops steaming. It should take about 5 minutes.

5. Serve hot topped with some tart jam, apple sauce, onion chip dip, or sour cream.

American Style Gluten-Free Frittatas

Ingredients

- 2 potatoes, peeled and cubed

- 1 1/2 teaspoons vegetable oil

- 1/4 onions, sliced

- 4 eggs, beaten

- Salt, to taste

- Pepper, to taste

- 5 cups cubed ham

- 1/4 cup cheddar cheese, shredded

Method

1. Add salt and water to a large pot, and bring to a boil. Add in the potatoes, and cook for about 5 minutes or until the potatoes are tender yet firm. Drain the water, and set the potatoes aside to cool.

2. Crank up your oven to 350 degrees F (175 degrees C), and let it preheat for at least 20 minutes.

3. Add the oil to a large cast-iron skillet, and heat it over a medium flame. Add in the onions, and cook on a medium-low flame, occasionally stirring until the onions are soft.

4. Add in the eggs, ham, drained potatoes, salt, and pepper. Continue cooking for 5 minutes or until the eggs are cooked on the bottom. Top the frittata with the shredded cheddar cheese, and place the skillet in the preheated oven till the cheese completely melts and the eggs are completely firm. This should take about 10 minutes.

5. Serve hot.

Gluten-Free Banana Bread

Ingredients

- 1 1/2 cups ripe bananas

- 1/4 cup melted butter

- 1/2 (15 ounce) can garbanzo beans (chickpeas), drained and rinsed

- 1/4 cup chopped pitted dates

- 2 tablespoons honey

- 1/4 cup almond flour

- 2 eggs

- 1/2 teaspoon grated fresh ginger

- 1/2 teaspoon baking soda

- 1/2 teaspoon ground cinnamon

- 1/2 teaspoon vanilla extract

- 1/4 teaspoon salt

Method

1. Crank up your oven to 350 degrees F (175 degrees C), and let it preheat for at least 20 minutes. Spray a large loaf pan with some oil, and set aside.

2. Blend together the bananas, chickpeas, almond flour, dates, and butter in a food processor or blender until smooth. Add in eggs, and whisk well.

3. Stir in the ginger, vanilla extract, honey, baking soda, cinnamon, and salt, and mix well until well combined. Do not over mix.

4. Pour the batter into the greased loaf plan.

5. Place the pan in the preheated oven, and bake for about an hour or until the bread turns golden brown and a knife inserted in the center of the loaf comes out clean.

6. Cool in the pan for about 20 minutes before slicing.

7. Serve warm.

Delicious Gluten-Free Homemade Fudge

Ingredients

- 2 (1 ounce) squares unsweetened chocolate, melted and cooled

- 3 ounces cream cheese, softened

- 1/4 teaspoon vanilla extract

- 1/8 teaspoon salt

- 2 cups confectioners' sugar, sifted

- 2/3 cup chopped walnuts

Method

1. Line a 4 by 4 inch dish with some foil. Spray some oil over it.

2. In a medium-sized mixing bowl, beat the cream cheese until it is smooth and no lumps remain.

3. Add in salt and vanilla extract, and beat until incorporated.

4. Add in the confectioners' sugar, a few teaspoons at a time, and continue beating until smooth.

5. Add in the melted chocolate, and mix well.

6. Gently fold in the walnuts.

7. Spread the prepared mix into the foil-lined pan, and chill in the refrigerator for an hour.

8. Cut into pieces, and serve cold.

Gluten-Free Peanut Butter Cookies

Ingredients

- 4 cups peanut butter

- 4 cups white sugar

- 2 3/4 cups chopped pecans (optional)

- 8 eggs, beaten

- 4 cups semi-sweet chocolate chips (optional)

Method

1. Crank up your oven to 350 degrees F (175 degrees C), and let it preheat for at least 20 minutes.

2. Combine the peanut butter, sugar, and eggs together in a large mixing bowl, and whisk until well combined. Add in the pecans and chocolate chips, if desired, and mix well.

3. Spoon the prepared dough onto the prepared cookie sheet.

4. Place the cookie sheet into the oven, and bake for about 10 to 12 minutes or until the cookies are lightly browned. Let the cookies cool on the cookie sheets for about 20 minutes.

5. Serve immediately, or store in an airtight box.

Gluten-Free Cream Cheese and Green Grape Salad

Ingredients

- 8 pounds seedless green grapes

- 2 (8 ounce) containers sour cream

- 2 (8 ounce) packages cream cheese

- 1 cup white sugar

- 1/2 pound pecans, chopped

- 2 teaspoons vanilla extract

- 4 tablespoons brown sugar

Method

1. Wash and dry the grapes.

2. In a bowl, combine the cream cheese, sugar, sour cream, and vanilla. Blend well until the mix is smooth and has no lumps in it.

3. Add the grapes, and mix well until well incorporated.

4. Add in the pecans and brown sugar, and mix well.

5. Chill in the refrigerator for a couple of hours.

6. Serve chilled.

Gluten-Free Chocolate Pudding with Almond Milk

Ingredients

- 2 cups white sugar, or to taste

- 2/3 cup cornstarch

- 1 cup unsweetened cocoa powder

- 1/2 teaspoon salt (optional)

- 2 teaspoons butter (optional)

- 6 cups unsweetened almond milk

- 2 teaspoons vanilla extract (optional)

Method

1. Combine the sugar, cornstarch, cocoa powder, and sugar in a saucepan. Add in about ½ cup of almond milk, and whisk well until smooth and frothy. Continue adding ½ cup of almond milk at a time, and whisk well between additions until the mixture is smooth and foamy.

2. Heat the saucepan over a medium-high flame and cook well while stirring constantly. Continue mixing until the mixture starts simmering and starts thickening up. This should take about 5 minutes.

3. Take the saucepan off the heat and mix in the butter. Whisk well until the butter has melted and the mix becomes smooth.

4. Divide the prepared mix into serving bowls, and chill for at least 30 minutes.

5. Serve chilled.

No-Bake Gluten-Free Coconut Chocolate Cookies

Ingredients

- 1/4 cup margarine

- 1 1/2 cups quick-cooking oats

- 1 cup white sugar

- 1/2 cup sweetened flaked coconut

- 1/4 cup unsweetened cocoa powder

- 1/4 cup milk

Method

1. Line a baking sheet with some parchment paper.

2. Mix the oats and sweetened flaked coconut until well combined.

3. Add the sugar, milk, cocoa powder, and margarine together in a heavy-bottomed saucepan. Heat over a medium flame, and mix well until smooth.

4. Bring the mix to a boil, and cook for 2 to 3 minutes while stirring constantly.

5. Pour the mix over the oat and coconut mix, and mix well to coat.

6. Dole out spoonfuls of the mixture on the prepared baking sheet. Set aside to cool and harden.

7. Store in an airtight container away from direct sunlight in a cool and dry place.

Chapter 18: Gluten-Free Recipes

In this segment, you will find several gluten-free recipes to help you kick-start your journey of going gluten-free and living a healthier life!

Breakfast Recipes

A lot of people skip breakfast, stating that they don't have time or that they really cannot eat in the morning. This is an extremely wrong attitude that should be changed as soon as possible!

Breakfast is one of the most important meals of the day, and it has to be your heaviest meal. Breakfast provides you with much-needed energy to go through the day, and if you skip it, you will feel lethargic and lazy!

Crustless Quiche

Ingredients

- 4 eggs, beaten
- ¼ cup milk
- ¼ teaspoon salt, or to taste
- ¼ teaspoon garlic powder

- ½ tablespoon olive oil

- ¼ cup green bell pepper, diced

- ¼ cup red bell pepper, diced

- ¼ cup corn kernels

- ¼–½ cup cheddar cheese, shredded

- ½ tablespoon honey mustard

- 1 tablespoon tapioca flour

- 1/8 teaspoon pepper, or to taste

- 1/8 teaspoon onion powder

Method

1. Turn up your oven to 350 degrees F (175 degrees C), and let it preheat for at least 20 minutes.

2. Lightly spray a 6-inch pie plate or cast-iron skillet with some cooking spray.

3. Pour the oil into a saucepan, and heat over a medium-high flame until the oil is heated. Add the bell peppers to the hot oil, and cook until they are a bit tender.

4. Turn off the heat, and stir in the corn kernels. Let it cool until the eggs are whisked.

5. Add eggs, milk, and honey mustard into a mixing bowl, and whisk well.

6. Whisk in the tapioca flour, garlic powder, salt, onion powder, and pepper. Add the bell pepper mixture into the bowl of eggs, and stir the mixture until well combined.

7. Add cheese and stir. Spoon the mixture into the pie plate. Scatter some more cheese on top. This is optional.

8. Pop the pie plate into the preheated oven, and bake for about 30 minutes or until the top of the quiche is evenly light brown.

9. Leave to cool for 5 minutes before serving.

10. Cut into 4 equal wedges and serve.

Scrambled Egg Tacos

Ingredients

- 1 tablespoon olive oil
- ¼ teaspoon cumin seeds
- Salt to taste
- ½ tablespoon fresh lemon juice
- 4 yellow corn tortillas
- ½ can (from a 15 ounce can) black beans, rinsed
- 2 small cloves garlic, peeled and minced
- Pepper to taste
- 2 cups baby spinach
- 4 large eggs
- ½ tablespoon water

Suggested Toppings (Optional)

- Queso fresco, crumbled
- Sour cream
- Chopped cilantro

Method

1. Pour half the oil into a saucepan, and heat over a medium-high flame until the oil is heated.

2. Add cumin seeds and garlic, and stir for a few seconds until fragrant and garlic turns light brown. Add beans and stir. Sprinkle salt and pepper to taste.

3. Stir in the spinach, and turn off the heat. Keep tossing until spinach wilts. Add lemon juice, and toss once again.

4. Combine water, eggs, pepper, and salt in a bowl. Whisk well.

5. Pour remaining oil into a nonstick skillet, and heat over a medium-high flame until the oil is heated.

6. Pour the egg mixture into the skillet, and stir often until the eggs are scrambled and soft-cooked or to your preference. Turn off the heat.

7. Heat the tortillas directly over the flame on your stovetop.

8. Divide the bean mixture among the tortillas. The same procedure goes with the scrambled eggs.

9. Sprinkle queso fresco and cilantro over the scrambled eggs. Drizzle some sour cream on top and serve.

Arianna Brooks

Mushrooms, Tomato, Bacon, and Cheddar Omelet

Ingredients

- 4 large eggs

- 6 large egg whites

- Pepper to taste

- 4 cups mushrooms, sliced

- 1 ounce cheddar cheese, sliced

- 4 green onions, sliced, divided

- 4 medium tomatoes, chopped

- 4 slices turkey bacon, cooked and chopped

Method

1. Whisk together eggs, whites, and pepper in a bowl.

2. Spray some cooking spray in a nonstick pan, and heat over a medium-high flame until the pan is heated.

3. Once the pan is hot, cook the mushrooms until brown and some liquid from the mushrooms is released in the pan.

4. Next, place the tomatoes into the ,pan along with most of the green onions, and cook for a few minutes until

slightly soft and the green onions wilt. Transfer the mixture into a bowl.

5. Spray some more cooking spray into the pan, and place it over a medium-low flame.

6. Pour half the egg mixture into the pan, and cook the omelet until eggs are set, making sure not to stir the eggs.

7. Spread half of the mushroom mixture on half of the omelet. Scatter half of the bacon and half of the cheese over the mushroom mixture. Fold the other half of the omelet over the filling. Remove the omelet and place on a plate.

8. Repeat the procedure (steps 5–7) to make the other omelet.

9. Sprinkle the remaining green onion on top and serve.

Oat Waffles

Ingredients

- ¾ cup gluten-free oat flour
- ¼ teaspoon salt
- 6 tablespoons milk of your choice, at room temperature
- 1 large egg
- ½ teaspoon vanilla extract
- 1 teaspoon baking powder
- 1/8 teaspoon ground cinnamon (optional)
- 2 ½ tablespoons coconut oil or unsalted butter, melted
- 1 tablespoon maple
- 1 tablespoon maple syrup

Suggested Toppings

- Maple syrup
- Whipped cream
- Nut butter
- Berries
- Any other toppings of your choice

Method

1. In a mixing bowl, combine baking powder, oat flour, cinnamon, and salt. Make sure they are well combined.

2. Combine coconut oil, milk, eggs, vanilla, and maple syrup in a microwave-safe bowl. Make sure they are well combined.

3. Place the bowl in a microwave, and heat the mixture (about 20 seconds) until the coconut oil melts and the mixture is smooth and well combined. Pour into the bowl of dry ingredients, and stir until the batter is incorporated. You may find a few lumps, but that is okay.

4. Set the batter aside for 10 minutes.

5. Set up your waffle maker, and let it preheat at medium-high for at least 10 minutes. Stir the batter lightly.

6. Spray the waffle iron with cooking spray, and pour 1/3 of the batter into the waffle maker. Follow the manufacturer's instructions, and cook the waffle to the desired doneness.

7. Remove the waffle, and keep warm in an oven if desired, or serve right away with suggested toppings.

8. Make the remaining 2 waffles in a similar manner (steps 6–7).

Layered Chia Pudding with Strawberry Fig Compote

Ingredients

For Pudding

- 6 tablespoons chia seeds

- 1 teaspoon vanilla extract

- 2 cups unsweetened almond milk

- 2 teaspoons raw honey, pure maple syrup, or stevia drops

For Compote

- 6 dried figs, finely chopped

- 1 cup fresh strawberries, sliced

For in-between layers

- 2 tablespoons natural almond butter

- 2 teaspoons raw honey

- 2 tablespoons unsweetened coconut, toasted lightly

Method

1. To make the pudding: Combine chia seeds, vanilla extract, almond milk, and sweetener in a bowl and stir.

2. Cover and chill for about an hour or two.

3. To make the compote: Place the figs and strawberries in a saucepan, and heat over a medium flame until the mixture comes to a light simmer. Mash with a potato masher as it cooks.

4. Lower the flame a bit, and cook for a couple of minutes. Turn off the heat, and transfer into a bowl.

5. Chill for about 20 minutes or until slightly thick.

6. To assemble: Take 2 mason jars, and spoon some pudding into the jars. Next, spoon some compote. Spoon some more pudding. Drizzle some honey and almond butter. Scatter some toasted coconut.

7. Repeat these layers until all the pudding and compote are used up.

8. You can serve right away or chill until use.

Breakfast Tofu Scramble

Ingredients

- 8 ounces extra-firm tofu, crumbled

- 1 medium onion, diced

- ½ cup chopped mushrooms

- 2 small cloves garlic, minced

- ¼ cup red bell pepper, diced

- ¼ cup green bell pepper, diced

- Pepper to taste

- 1/8 teaspoon turmeric powder

- ¼ teaspoon ground cumin

- Salt to taste

Method

1. Pour about 2 tablespoons of water into a skillet, and heat over a medium flame until the water is heated. You can use a tablespoon of oil instead of water.

2. Add onion and cook until pink. Stir in the garlic, and cook for about a minute or until you get a nice aroma.

3. Stir in the bell peppers and mushrooms. Sprinkle some more water if the vegetables are getting stuck to the bottom of the pan.

4. Once the vegetables are tender, add turmeric and stir for 5–6 seconds.

5. Stir in the tofu, cumin, salt, and pepper. Heat thoroughly, stirring often.

6. You can serve as it is or over corn tortillas or gluten-free bread slices.

Toasted Coconut Amaranth Porridge

Ingredients

- ¼ cup unsweetened coconut flakes

- 1 ½ cups water

- ½ cup coconut milk

- Toasted, slivered almonds (optional)

- ½ cup amaranth

- 1/8 teaspoon kosher salt

- Honey to taste

- 1 ½ cups water

- ½ cup coconut milk

Method

1. Turn up your oven to 350 degrees F (175 degrees C), and let it preheat for 5 minutes.

2. Line a baking sheet with foil. Spread coconut on the baking sheet. Place the baking sheet in the oven, and toast for a few minutes until light golden brown or golden brown as per your preference. Leave to cool on your countertop.

3. Pour water into a saucepan, and heat over a medium flame until the water comes to a boil.

4. Stir in amaranth and salt. Cook covered on low flame until dry. Turn off the heat. Add coconut milk and coconut flakes and stir.

5. Add honey if desired.

6. Divide into 2 bowls. Garnish with almonds and serve.

Hot Water Cornbread

Ingredients

- ½ cup cornmeal

- ½ teaspoon white sugar

- 6 tablespoons boiling water

- ½ teaspoon salt

- ½ tablespoon shortening

- Oil to fry, as required

- Honey or maple syrup or any other syrup of your choice

Method

1. Add cornmeal, sugar, and salt into a mixing bowl, and stir well.

2. Pour boiling water, and add the shortening. Mix well until the shortening has melted completely.

3. Pour oil into a skillet such that it is about ½–1 inch in height from the bottom of the pan. Let the oil heat to 375 degrees F (190 degrees C).

4. Meanwhile, make 12 equal portions of the cornmeal dough, and shape them into balls. Flatten each ball.

5. When the oil is heated, drop a few of the flattened dough carefully, and cook until golden brown all over.

6. Remove with a slotted spoon, and place on a plate lined with paper towels.

7. Fry the remaining dough balls in batches.

8. Serve drizzled with maple syrup or honey or any other syrup of your choice.

Gluten-Free Pancakes

Ingredients

- ½ cup rice flour

- 3 tablespoons potato starch

- ½ packet sugar substitute or sugar to taste

- ¼ teaspoon baking soda

- 1 ½ tablespoons tapioca flour

- 2 tablespoons dry buttermilk powder

- ¼ teaspoon salt

- ¾ teaspoon baking powder

- ¼ teaspoon xanthan gum

- 1 ½ tablespoons canola oil

- 1 egg

- 1 cup water

Method

1. Combine all the dry ingredients in a bowl: rice flour, potato starch, tapioca flour, sugar substitute, buttermilk powder, baking soda, baking powder, xanthan gum, and salt.

2. Add water, egg, and oil, and stir until well combined. You may find the batter slightly lumpy. Let it rest for 5 minutes.

3. Stir once again.

4. Place a griddle or pan over medium flame. Grease it with some cooking spray. Pour 1/5 of the batter into the skillet. In a minute or so, you will see bubbles on top of the pancake. Cook until the underside is golden brown. Flip sides, and cook the other side as well.

5. Remove onto a plate and serve with syrup or toppings of your choice.

6. Cook the remaining pancakes similarly.

Granola Bars

Ingredients

- 6 tablespoons natural peanut butter or any other nut butter of your choice

- 1/8 teaspoon ground cinnamon

- 1 cup gluten-free rolled oats

- 3 tablespoons pure maple syrup or agave syrup

- 1/8 teaspoon salt

Method

1. Place a sheet of parchment paper in a small, square baking pan (about 4–5 inches).

2. Add peanut butter and maple syrup into a microwave-safe bowl. Place the bowl in the microwave, and cook on high for about a minute or until well heated.

3. Stir until smooth and well combined. You can also place the ingredients in a pan, and cook on the stovetop over a low flame.

4. Stir in cinnamon and salt. Once well combined, stir in the oats.

5. Transfer the mixture into the prepared baking pan. Press it well onto the bottom of the pan, and let it chill for an hour.

6. Cut into 4 equal slices and serve.

Gluten-Free Irish Soda Bread

Ingredients

- 1/2 cup buttermilk
- 3/4 cup white rice flour
- 1/2 egg
- 1/4 cup tapioca flour
- 1/2 teaspoon baking powder
- 1/2 teaspoon baking soda
- 1/4 cup white sugar
- 1/2 teaspoon salt

Method

1. Turn up your oven to oven to 350 degrees F (175 degrees C), and allow it to preheat for at least 20 minutes. Lightly spray a 5-inch round cake pan with some cooking spray, and lightly flour it with some white rice flour.

2. Sieve together the white rice flour, white sugar, tapioca flour, baking powder, baking soda, and salt in a large-sized mixing bowl.

3. In another medium-sized bowl, whisk the egg until light and frothy. Pour the buttermilk onto the frothy eggs, and whisk to combine. Do not over whisk.

4. Create a small hole in the center of the dry ingredients by pushing them to the sides of the bowl. Pour the egg and buttermilk mixture in the center of the hole, and slowly start pushing a small quantity of the dry ingredients from the side to the center, mixing well after each addition. Repeat until all the dry ingredients have been combined with the wet ingredients.

5. Pour the prepared batter into the greased and floured cake pan. Pop into the preheated oven, and bake at 350 degrees F (175 degrees C) for about 60 minutes or until a skewer inserted in the center of the bread comes out clean and batter-free.

6. Carefully remove the pan from the oven, and allow the pan to cool for about 10 minutes on a wire rack. Remove the bread from the cake pan, and wrap it in aluminum foil or plastic wrap. Allow the bread to stand for about 8 hours or overnight.

7. Slice and serve with a side of your favorite jam, jelly, or fruit – this bread tastes delicious with them all!

Gluten-Free Ham and Cheese Quiche with Hash Brown Base

Ingredients

- 6 cups russet potatoes, grated
- 1 cup heavy whipping cream
- 2 cups cooked diced ham
- 2/3 cup butter, melted (can use margarine instead)
- 4 eggs
- 2 cups cheese, shredded

Method

1. Turn up your oven to oven to 425 degrees F (220 degrees C), and allow it to preheat for at least 20 minutes.

2. Using your hands, pick up fistfuls of the shredded potatoes, and squeeze until all the excess moisture present in the potatoes is removed.

3. Place these squeezed out potatoes in a bowl, and add the melted butter (or melted margarine) to the potatoes. Mix well to combine.

4. Empty the above mixture into a 10-inch pan pie, and lightly press it into the bottom of the ungreased pan.

5. Pop pan into the preheated oven, and bake for about 25 to 30 minutes at 425 degrees F (220 degrees C).

6. Once the potatoes are a beautiful golden color, carefully take the pan out of the oven. Do not turn the oven off.

7. Place the ham and cheese on the prepared potato base.

8. In a small bowl, whisk the eggs until frothy. Add in the heavy whipping cream, and mix well. Pour this egg and cream mixture over the ham and cheese.

9. Return the pan to the oven and bake for another 30 minutes at 425 degrees F (220 degrees C) or until the quiche has perfectly set and is firm to touch.

10. Allow the pan to cool for a few minutes before removing the quiche from the pan.

11. Cut into pieces and serve hot!

Delectable Gluten-Free Rice and Tapioca Flour Pancakes

Ingredients

- 1/2 cup rice flour

- 8 teaspoons potato starch

- 4 1/2 teaspoons tapioca flour

- 1/2 packet sugar substitute

- 2 tablespoons dry buttermilk powder

- 3/4 teaspoon baking powder

- 1/4 teaspoon salt

- 1/4 teaspoon baking soda

- 1 egg

- 1/4 teaspoon xanthan gum

- 1 cup water

- 4 1/2 teaspoons canola oil

Method

1. Sieve the rice flour, potato starch, tapioca flour, sugar substitute, dry buttermilk powder, baking powder, salt,

baking soda, and xanthan gum together in a larger mixing bowl.

2. In a small bowl, whisk the egg until light and frothy. Pour in the canola oil, and whisk until combined.

3. Pour the egg and oil mixture into the dry ingredients, and mix well until the batter is well blended and there are not too many lumps in it.

4. Place a large skillet or griddle on a stove, and heat over a medium-high flame. Add in just enough oil to grease.

5. Pour about 3 tablespoons of the batter on the hot skillet or griddle, and ensure that the batter is well spread. Cook until the batter starts bubbling.

6. Flip the pancake over, and keep cooking until the other side is well browned. Repeat with the remaining batter.

7. Serve hot, doused in maple syrup or with a side of some whipped cream or your favorite fresh fruits!

Appetizer Recipes

Who says you can't plan a party while being on a strict diet? Appetizers are the life of a party – after all, no one came to see you; they just came for the free food! However, sadly, most appetizers are loaded with gluten, often making it almost impossible to plan a gluten-free menu! Fret not. These delicious tidbits will add another level of deliciousness to your party, and not one person will be able to guess that these dishes are 100% gluten-free!

Caprese Salad Bites

Ingredients

- 24 cherry tomatoes or grape tomatoes

- 7.5 ounces mozzarella cheese, cut into 12 equal square pieces

- 12 fresh basil leaves, halved

- 1 ½ tablespoons rosemary balsamic dressing

Method

1. Take 12 small wooden skewers. Thread a cherry tomato, a basil leaf, a mozzarella piece, basil, and a cherry tomato on each skewer. Fold the basil half while threading onto the skewers.

2. Place the skewers on a plate. Drizzle rosemary balsamic dressing over the skewers.

3. Chill if desired, or serve right away.

Mexican Street Corn Dip

Ingredients

- 2 teaspoons canola oil

- 2 jalapeño peppers, deseeded and finely chopped

- ½ cup Mexican crema or sour cream

- 2 teaspoons chili powder

- ¼ teaspoon cayenne pepper

- 2 packages (14.5 ounces each) corn tortilla chips, to serve

- 4 2/3 cups fresh or frozen corn kernels thaw if frozen

- ½ cup mayonnaise

- 4 tablespoons lime juice

- 1 ½ cups crumbled queso fresco, divided

- Chopped cilantro to garnish

Method

1. Turn up your oven to 350 degrees F (175 degrees C), and let it preheat for at least 20 minutes.

2. Pour the oil into a saucepan, and heat over a medium-high flame until the oil is heated.

3. Stir in the corn kernels and jalapeño. Stir until the underside of the kernels is light brown. It should take about 3–4 minutes.

4. Give it a good stir, and let it cook undisturbed for about 3 minutes or until light brown on the underside.

5. Turn off the heat, and add mayonnaise, lime juice, 1 cup queso fresco, Mexican crema, and chili powder, and stir well.

6. Spoon the mixture into a baking dish. You can also use a glass pie pan. Scatter remaining queso fresco and cayenne over the corn mixture.

7. Pop the pie plate into the preheated oven, and bake for about 15–20 minutes or until the cheese melts.

8. Leave to cool for 5 minutes before serving.

9. Sprinkle cilantro on top. This is to be served with tortilla chips.

Zucchini Pizza Bites

Ingredients

- 2 large zucchinis, cut into 1 inch thick, round slices

- Salt to taste

- 6 tablespoons part-skim mozzarella cheese, shredded

- 1 tablespoon parmesan cheese, finely grated

- ¼ teaspoon pepper or to taste

- ¼ cup low-sodium marinara sauce

- 8 slices pepperoni

Method

1. Turn up your oven to 350 degrees F (175 degrees C), and let it preheat for at least 20 minutes.

2. Take zucchini slices, and place them on a baking sheet. Season with salt and pepper.

3. Pop the baking sheet into the preheated oven, and bake for about 15–20 minutes or until zucchini is slightly soft.

4. Spread marinara sauce on the zucchini slices. Sprinkle mozzarella on the zucchini slices. Place pepperoni slices on top.

5. Set the rack about 8 inches below the heating element in the oven.

6. Turn the oven to broil mode. Broil for a few minutes until the cheese is brown at a few spots.

7. Garnish with parmesan on top.

Egg BLTs

Ingredients

- 3 large eggs, hard-boiled, peeled, and halved crosswise

- ½ cup baby spinach

- 2 tablespoons avocado, mashed

- 1 teaspoon lemon juice

- Pepper to taste

- 2 slices thick-cut bacon, cooked cut into thirds

- 1 small tomato, thinly sliced

- 1 tablespoon mayonnaise

- Salt to taste

Method

1. Place 2 bacon slices on each of the 3 egg halves. Place spinach and tomato slices over the bacon.

2. Add avocado, lemon juice, mayonnaise, salt, and pepper in a bowl, and mix well. Smear this mixture over the cut part of the remaining 3 egg halves. Cover the sandwich with these egg halves, with the cut part over the tomato slices.

3. Insert toothpicks to keep the sandwiches in place. Sprinkle pepper on top and serve.

Loaded Sheet-Pan Nachos

Ingredients

- 1 teaspoon extra-virgin olive oil

- ½ medium red onion, diced

- ½ package (from a 13 ounces package) corn tortilla chips

- 2 tablespoons pickled jalapeños

- ½ medium green bell pepper, diced

- ¼ teaspoon salt or to taste

- 4 ounces Mexican cheese blend or cheddar cheese, shredded

Suggested Toppings

- A handful fresh cilantro, chopped

- Sliced scallion

- Sour cream

- Salsa Verde

- Diced avocado

Method

1. Turn up your oven to 400 degrees F (205 degrees C), and let it preheat for at least 20 minutes.

2. Pour the oil into a saucepan, and heat over a medium-high flame until the oil is heated.

3. Once the oil is hot, add onion, bell pepper, and salt, and stir-fry for a couple of minutes until slightly tender. Turn off the heat.

4. Spread half the chips on a rimmed baking sheet, without the chips overlapping each other.

5. Scatter half the bell pepper mixture over the chips, followed by about 1 ¼ ounce cheese.

6. Spread the remaining chips over the cheese layer, followed by the remaining bell pepper mixture and cheese. Scatter jalapeños on top.

7. Pop the baking sheet into the preheated oven, and bake for about 10 minutes or until cheese melts and is brown at a few spots.

8. Top with the suggested toppings and serve.

Tropical Snack Mix

Ingredients

- ½ cup cashews, roasted and lightly salted

- ½ cup unsweetened coconut flakes

- ½ cup unsweetened dried pineapple, chopped

- ½ cup unsweetened dried mango, chopped

Method

1. Add nuts, coconut, dried pineapple, and mango into an airtight container and toss well. Seal the container, and store it at room temperature. It can last for 2 weeks.

Buffalo Chicken Wings

Ingredients

- 12 chicken wings, discard tips, and cut the wings into 2 halves from the joint

- ½ tablespoon distilled white vinegar

- Salt to taste

- 2 tablespoons butter

- Pepper to taste

- 2 ½ tablespoons hot pepper sauce

- Vegetable oil to fry, as required

Method

1. Pour enough oil into a deep skillet or deep fryer (at least 3–4 inches in height from the bottom of the pan). Let the oil heat to 375 degrees F (190 degrees C).

2. Add chicken wings in batches, and cook until the desired doneness is achieved.

3. Remove chicken with a slotted spoon and place on a plate lined with layers of paper towels.

4. Add butter into a skillet and heat over a medium flame until butter melts.

5. Add hot pepper sauce, salt, pepper, and vinegar. Add the fried chicken into the skillet, and stir until the sauce mixture is well-coated on the chicken wings.

6. Simmer for a few minutes and serve.

Turkey Meatballs

Ingredients

- 4 ounces chicken sausage, discard casings

- 6 ounces ground turkey

- 1 ½ tablespoons fresh basil, minced

- 1 teaspoon garlic or garlic powder, minced

- ½ teaspoon kosher salt

- 1 small egg, lightly beaten

- 1/3 cup gluten-free breadcrumbs

- 1 ½ tablespoons milk

- 2 tablespoons parmesan cheese, grated

- ¼ teaspoon pepper

Method

1. Turn up your oven to 350 degrees F (175 degrees C), and let it preheat for at least 10 minutes. Prepare a baking sheet by lining it with parchment paper.

2. Add sausage, turkey, basil, garlic, salt, egg, breadcrumbs, milk, parmesan, and pepper into a bowl, and mix with a fork until just incorporated.

3. Divide the mixture into 20 equal portions, and shape into balls of about 1 ¼ inch diameter. Place on the baking sheet. You can also scoop the mixture with a spoon and drop it on the baking sheet.

4. Pop the baking sheet in the oven, and bake for about 30 minutes until light brown. The internal temperature of the meatballs should read 165 degrees F (74 degrees F).

Easy Gluten-Free Guacamole

Ingredients

- 1/2 small onion
- Pepper, to taste
- 1 avocado
- 1/2 small ripe tomato
- 1/2 clove garlic
- Salt, to taste
- Juice of ½ lime

Method

1. Peel the avocado, and smash the pulp in a smooth paste in a small bowl.

2. Chop the onion finely into small ¼ inch cubes, and place in the bowl with the mashed avocado pulp. Mince the garlic finely, and add to the avocado pulp. Mix well.

3. Add in the lime juice, pepper, and salt and taste. Adjust seasoning accordingly.

4. Dice the ripe tomato, and put into the bowl. Mix with a light hand so that the tomato doesn't get mushed.

5. Cover the bowl with a plastic wrap, and place in the refrigerator. Chill for at least 8 hours or overnight.

6. Serve chilled with carrot, cucumber, and beetroot sticks.

Buttery Basil and Lemon Shrimp

Ingredients

- 6 pounds fresh shrimp, skinned, and deveined
- 1 cup fresh basil leaves, minced finely
- 1/4 cup Dijon mustard
- 1/4 cup olive oil
- Juice of 3 lemons
- 1/2 cup butter, melted
- 6 cloves garlic, crushed
- Salt, to taste
- White pepper, to taste
- Skewers

Method

1. Combine the olive oil and melted butter in a small dish or a shallow bowl. Add the minced basil leaves, Dijon mustard, lemon juice, and crushed garlic to the butter and olive oil mix, and mix well to combine. Taste and season accordingly with white pepper and salt.

2. Add the peeled and deveined shrimp to the marinade mix, and toss well so that the shrimp gets coated with the marinade mix. Cover the bowl with a plastic wrap, and let the shrimp marinate for at least 2 hours or more.

3. While the shrimp marinates, turn your grill up to high heat, and allow it to preheat for at least 30 minutes. If you are using wooden skewers, soak the skewers in some warm, lightly salted water for at least 30 minutes.

4. Drain the shrimp from the marinade, and get rid of the extra marinade.

5. Thread the drained shrimp on to the prepared skewers. Lightly spray the grate of the grill with some cooking spray, and place the prepared shrimp skewers on the grill.

6. Cook the shrimp for at least 4 minutes on each side or until the shrimps turn opaque.

7. Serve hot with a condiment of your choice.

Arianna Brooks

Garlicky Stuffed Portobello Mushroom Caps

Ingredients

- 1/2 cup balsamic vinegar
- 6 Portobello mushrooms
- 1 medium onion, chopped
- 1/2 cup canola oil
- 8 cloves garlic, minced

Method

1. Clean the mushrooms, and get rid of all the dirt. Remove the stems of the mushrooms, and save them for use later.

2. Place the mushroom caps on a flat surface, like a plate or a baking sheet, with the gill side of the mushroom facing upwards.

3. Combine the balsamic vinegar, chopped onion, canola oil, and minced garlic together in a small mixing bowl. Chill for at least 15 minutes in the refrigerator.

4. Spoon the mixture into the Portobello mushroom caps, and cover the mushrooms with a soft muslin cloth. Let the mushrooms sit for at least an hour.

5. Preheat the grill on a high flame for at least 20 to 25 minutes. Place the stuffed mushroom caps on the hot grill, and grill for at least 10 minutes or until done.

6. Serve immediately with a condiment of your choice.

Lunch or Dinner Recipes

Your lunch and dinner are the main components of your day and consist of the food that you eat to satiate yourself and provide your body with much-needed nutrition. A lot of times, while on a highly restrictive diet like the gluten-free diet, you find yourself at your wits end wondering what to cook and what to eat. To help you get started, we have provided you with some recipes that you can easily make in the confines of your kitchen in a very short time!

Greek Salmon Bowl

Ingredients

- ½ pound salmon fillets

- Pepper to taste

- ¾ cup + 2 tablespoons water

- 1 ½ tablespoons lemon juice

- 2 small cloves garlic, peeled and minced

- ½ medium tomato, deseeded and diced

- 2 cups pitted, sliced kalamata olives

- ¼ teaspoon salt or to taste

- 4 ounces string beans, trimmed and cut into 1 inch pieces

- 6 tablespoons quinoa, rinsed

- 1 tablespoon olive oil

- 1 teaspoon fresh oregano + extra to garnish or use ¼ teaspoon dried oregano, chopped

- 2 tablespoons feta cheese, crumbled

Method

1. Turn up your oven to 400 degrees F (205 degrees C), and let it preheat for at least 20 minutes.

2. Place a sheet of foil on a baking sheet. Lay the salmon fillets on the baking sheet. Season with a bit of salt and pepper.

3. Pop the baking sheet in the oven, and bake for about 20 minutes or until cooked through.

4. Leave to cool for 5 minutes. Peel off the skin, and discard it. Cut salmon into bite-size pieces.

5. Pour some water into a saucepan, and place a steamer on top of it. Heat the saucepan on high flame until the water is bubbling.

6. Place the beans in the steamer, and cover with a lid. Steam the beans for about 5 minutes or until the beans are crisp and tender.

7. Put the beans under cold, running water, and let it drain.

8. To cook quinoa: Add quinoa and water into a saucepan, and heat over a high flame until it comes to a boil.

9. Lower the heat, and cook covered until nearly dry. Turn off the heat, and let it sit covered for 5 minutes. Using a fork, fluff the quinoa.

10. To make the dressing: Add garlic, lemon juice, oregano, oil, and a little salt into a bowl and whisk well.

11. To assemble: Place equal amounts of quinoa in 2 serving bowls. Divide equally the salmon, beans, feta, tomatoes, and olives among the bowls, and place over the quinoa.

12. Trickle the dressing, and sprinkle oregano on top.

13. Serve.

Chopped Salad with Chicken and Avocado-Buttermilk Dressing

Ingredients

For Avocado-Buttermilk Dressing

- ½ cup buttermilk

- 1 ½ tablespoons fresh herbs of your choice, minced

- ½ teaspoon salt

- ¼ ripe avocado, peeled and chopped

- ½ tablespoon rice vinegar

- ¼ teaspoon pepper, or to taste

For Salad

- 2 cups kale, chopped

- 1 cup broccoli florets, finely chopped

- ½ cup carrots, shredded

- 1 cup red cabbage, shredded

- 1 cup cooked chicken, shredded

- ¼ cup almonds, sliced and toasted

- ¼ cup red onions, finely chopped

- 3 tablespoons dried cranberries or cherries

Method

1. To make dressing: Blend together buttermilk, vinegar, herbs, avocado, and seasonings into a blender, and blend until smooth.

2. To make salad: Add vegetables, almonds, and cherries into a bowl, and toss well.

3. Pour dressing on top. Toss well and serve.

Shrimp Avocado Salad

Ingredients

For Salad

- ½ pound shrimp, peeled, deveined, and coarsely chopped

- 1 green onion, chopped

- ½ jalapeño pepper, deseeded and minced

- Cilantro, chopped

- 1 plum tomato, chopped

- 2 tablespoons red onion, finely chopped

- ½ Serrano pepper, deseeded and minced

- 1 ½ medium ripe avocados, peeled, pitted, and cubed

For Dressing

- 1 tablespoon lime juice

- 1 tablespoon olive oil

- 1 tablespoon seasoned rice vinegar

- ½ teaspoon adobo seasoning

To Serve

- Lime wedges

- Bibb lettuce leaves

Method

1. To make dressing: Whisk together lime juice, oil, seasoned rice vinegar, and adobo seasoning in a bowl. Set aside for a while for the flavors to meld.

2. To make salad: Add shrimp, green onion, red onion, tomato, and peppers into a bowl, and toss well.

3. Cover the bowl, and chill for an hour or two.

4. Add avocadoes just before serving. Toss gently.

5. To assemble: Place lettuce leaves on a serving platter. Fill the salad over the lettuce leaves. This is to be served with lime wedges.

Afghan Vegetable and Chickpea Soup (Tarkari)

Ingredients

- 1 teaspoon extra-virgin olive oil

- ½ small onion, diced

- 2 cups low-sodium vegetable broth

- 1/3 cup frozen corn

- ¼ teaspoon salt

- ¼ cup packed spinach, chopped

- ½ large carrot, diced

- 1 clove garlic, minced

- ½ can (from a 15 ounce can) chickpeas, drained and rinsed

- 1/3 cup frozen peas

- ¼ teaspoon pepper or to taste

- 3 fresh sprigs cilantro, to garnish

Method

1. Pour oil into a saucepan, and heat over a medium flame until the oil is hot.

2. Once oil is hot, stir in garlic, onion, and carrot, and cook until onion turns translucent.

3. Add chickpeas, peas, corn, broth, and seasonings and stir. When it comes to a boil, lower the flame and simmer for about 8–9 minutes.

4. Add spinach, and cook for a minute.

5. Ladle into soup bowls. Garnish with cilantro sprigs and serve.

Spiced Carrot and Lentil Soup

Ingredients

- 1 teaspoon cumin seeds

- 1 tablespoon olive oil

- 2 1/2 ounces split red lentils

- ¼ cup milk

- Chili flakes to taste

- Yogurt to garnish

- 10 1/2 ounces carrots, grated

- Salt to taste

- 2 cups vegetable stock

- Pepper to taste

Method

1. Add cumin and chili flakes into a saucepan, and roast over a medium flame. In about a minute, the cumin will begin to crackle. Set aside half the cumin and chili flakes in a bowl.

2. Add oil into the saucepan. Once oil is heated, add carrots, stock, lentils, and milk and stir.

3. When it begins to boil, lower the heat and cook covered until the lentils are soft.

4. Blend with an immersion blender until smooth.

5. Add salt and pepper to taste.

6. Divide into 2 soup bowls. Drizzle some yogurt on top. Garnish with the retained cumin seeds and chili flakes.

7. Serve as it is or over rice or gluten-free bread.

Creamy Cauliflower Soup

Ingredients

- 1 tablespoon salted butter

- ½ large head cauliflower, cut into florets

- 1 ½ stalks celery, sliced

- 2 cloves garlic, minced

- ½ teaspoon dried oregano

- 1 cup vegetable broth

- Salt to taste

- ½ tablespoon extra-virgin olive oil

- ½ white onion, diced

- 1 ½ carrots, diced

- 1 ½ stalks celery, sliced

- 2 cloves garlic, minced

- ½ teaspoon dried oregano

- ½ teaspoon dried thyme

- 1 tablespoon cornstarch

- Salt to taste

- 1 cup milk

- 1 cup vegetable broth

- Pepper to taste

Method

1. Add oil and butter into a soup pot, and heat over a medium-high flame until butter melts.

2. Once butter melts, add the vegetables and cook until slightly tender.

3. Stir in garlic, and cook for a few seconds until you get a nice aroma.

4. Add dried herbs and cornstarch, and constantly stir for about a minute.

5. Add milk and broth, stirring constantly. Keep stirring until it begins to boil.

6. Lower the flame, and simmer until the soup is thick. Add salt and pepper and stir.

7. Divide the soup into 3 bowls and serve.

Vegetable, Steak, and Eggs

Ingredients

- ½ pound beef skirt steak or flank steak

- 1 tablespoon butter or coconut oil, divided

- ½ medium yellow summer squash, halved lengthwise and cut into ¼ inch thick slices

- 3 cups baby spinach

- Pepper to taste

- 2 tablespoons parmesan cheese, shredded

- ½ teaspoon Montreal steak seasoning

- ½ medium zucchini halved lengthwise, cut into ¼ inch thick slices

- ½ medium red bell pepper, chopped

- Salt to taste

- 2 large eggs

Method

1. Sprinkle Montreal steak seasoning over the steak, and rub it well.

2. Set up your grill, and preheat it to medium-high heat for about 20 minutes. You can also broil it in an oven.

3. Place steak on the grill, and cook for about 5 minutes on each side for a medium steak. You may increase or decrease the cooking time, depending upon the doneness desired.

4. Once the steaks are cooked, transfer the steaks to your cutting board. Let it rest until the vegetables are cooked.

5. To cook vegetables: Add ½ tablespoon butter into a nonstick pan, and melt over a medium-high flame.

6. Once butter melts, add squash, zucchini, and bell pepper, and cook for a few minutes until vegetables are crisp and slightly tender.

7. Stir in spinach and seasonings. Cook for a couple of minutes until spinach wilts.

8. Transfer the vegetable mixture into 2 warm plates.

9. Add ½ tablespoon butter into the same pan. Once butter melts, crack the eggs into the pan, and cook the eggs the way you prefer.

10. Cut the steak into thin slices across the grain.

11. Top the vegetables with steak slices. Place an egg on top of each plate. Sprinkle a tablespoon of cheese on each plate and serve.

Chili Skillet

Ingredients

- ½ pound ground beef

- ¼ cup green bell pepper, chopped

- ½ can (from a 16 ounces can) kidney beans, rinsed and drained

- ¼ cup water

- ½ teaspoon dried oregano

- ¼ cup uncooked long grain rice

- ¼ cup sliced ripe olives

- 1 green onion, thinly sliced (optional)

- ½ cup chopped onion

- 2 small cloves garlic, peeled and minced

- ½ cup tomato juice

- 2 teaspoons chili powder

- ½ teaspoon salt

- ½ cup canned or frozen corn kernels

- ½ cup cheddar cheese or Monterey Jack cheese, shredded

Method

1. Add beef, garlic, bell pepper, and onion into a skillet, and cook over a medium flame until the meat is no longer pink.

2. Add water, oregano, rice, kidney beans, tomato juice, chili powder, and salt and stir.

3. Cover and cook on low heat until rice is cooked.

4. Add olives and corn, and continue cooking covered for another 5 minutes.

5. Scatter cheese on top, and cover once again. Cook until the cheese melts.

6. Garnish with green onions and serve.

Pork Tenderloin with Roasted Red Grapes and Cabbage

Ingredients

- 1 ½ tablespoons olive oil

- ¾ pound purple cabbage, cut into ½ inch wedges

- ¾ pound pork tenderloin, cut into 2 equal parts

- 2 sprigs fresh thyme, torn

- 1 shallot, halved

- ¼ cup red wine

- Salt to taste

- 1 cup red grapes

- Pepper to taste

Method

1. Turn up your oven to 450 degrees F (230 degrees C), and let it preheat for at least 15 minutes.

2. Grease a rimmed baking sheet with a tablespoon of oil.

3. Sprinkle thyme over the baking sheet, and lay the cabbage wedges and shallot halves on it in a single layer.

4. Place grapes over the cabbage. Season with salt and pepper.

5. Pop the baking sheet in the oven, and bake until shallots turn brown and cabbage, and grapes are slightly soft. Remove the baking sheet from the oven, and drizzle vinegar over the vegetables. Scrape the bottom of the baking sheet to remove any brown bits.

6. While the vegetables are roasting, add ½ tablespoon oil into a skillet, and heat until the oil is hot.

7. Sprinkle salt and pepper over the pork, and place it on the skillet. Cook until golden brown all over and cooked through inside.

8. Remove pork from the pan, and place it on your cutting board. Cool for about 8–9 minutes.

9. Slice the pork, and serve with roasted vegetables and grapes. Drizzle the vinegar from the baking sheet over the pork and roasted grapes and vegetables.

Tequila Lime Shrimp Zoodles

Ingredients

- 1 ½ tablespoons butter, divided
- 1 clove garlic, peeled and minced
- ¾ teaspoon grated lime zest + extra to serve
- ½ tablespoon olive oil
- 1 medium zucchini, trimmed
- Pepper to taste
- ½ shallot, minced
- 2 tablespoons tequila
- 1 tablespoon lime juice
- ½ pound uncooked shrimp, peeled and deveined
- ¼ teaspoon salt, or to taste
- 1/8 cup fresh parsley, minced

Method

1. Make noodles of the zucchini using a spiralizer or a julienne peeler.

2. Add butter into a heavy skillet, and heat over a medium flame. Once butter melts, add garlic and shallot, and sauté for a couple of minutes. Turn off the heat, and add lime juice and lime zest. Also, add tequila and stir.

3. Place it back over a medium flame, and cook until nearly dry.

4. Stir in shrimp, zucchini, remaining butter, and olive oil. Add salt and pepper to taste and stir. Stir occasionally.

5. Once the shrimp turns pink, turn off the heat. Garnish with parsley and lime zest and serve.

Cod with Herbed Pea Relish

Ingredients

For Cod

- ½ tablespoon olive oil
- Salt to taste
- 2 cod fillets (6 ounces each)

For Pea Relish

- ½ cup frozen green peas, thawed
- 1 tablespoon shallots, chopped
- 1 tablespoon lime juice
- Salt to taste
- 2 teaspoon fresh oregano, minced
- 1 tablespoon capers
- 1 tablespoon olive oil
- 1/8 teaspoon crushed red pepper or to taste

Method

1. To make relish: Add peas, shallots, lime juice, salt, oregano, capers, olive oil, and crushed red pepper into a bowl, and mix well. Cover and set aside until it is time to serve.

2. To cook the cod: Pour oil into a nonstick skillet, and heat over a medium-high flame until the oil is heated.

3. Sprinkle salt over the cod, and place it in the pan. Flip the fillets after 4 minutes. Cook for 4 minutes, and remove from the pan.

4. Serve cod with pea relish.

Sesame Chicken and Chili Lime Slaw

Ingredients

For Sesame Chicken

- 1 large egg white
- Salt to taste
- 2 chicken breasts (5 ounces each), boneless and skinless
- ½ tablespoon olive oil
- ¼ cup sesame seeds

For Chili Lime Slaw

- 2 tablespoons lime juice
- ½ teaspoon honey
- 10 ounces red cabbage, finely shredded
- ¼ cup fresh cilantro, chopped
- ½ tablespoon fresh ginger, grated
- ½ small red chili, thinly sliced
- 1 large carrot, coarsely grated
- Salt to taste
- Pepper to taste

Method

1. Turn up your oven to 450 degrees F (230 degrees C), and let it preheat for at least 15 minutes.

2. Place sesame seeds on a plate. Whisk together egg white and salt in a shallow bowl. Dunk the chicken breasts in this. Shake off any extra white from the chicken. Dredge the chicken in sesame seeds, and place on a plate.

3. Place a cast-iron skillet over a medium flame, and allow it to heat.

4. Pour oil into the skillet. Swirl the pan to spread the oil. Place chicken in the pan, and cook until golden brown on either side. Turn off the heat.

5. Shift the skillet into the oven, and roast for about 10 minutes or until well-cooked inside.

6. To make chili lime slaw: Add lime juice, honey, salt, chili, pepper, and ginger into a bowl, and whisk well.

7. Add cabbage and carrots, and toss well. Add cilantro, and toss once again.

8. Serve slaw with chicken.

Chicken with Stewed Peppers and Tomatoes

Ingredients

For Chicken

- 2 chicken breasts (6 ounces each), skinless and boneless
- Salt to taste
- ½ tablespoon paprika
- Pepper to taste
- ½ tablespoon olive oil

For Stewed Tomatoes and Peppers

- 1 small red onion, cut into ½ inch thick slices
- ¼ pound Campari or large cherry tomatoes, halved
- 1 red bell pepper, quartered and cut into ½ inch thick pieces crosswise
- 1 large clove garlic, thinly sliced

To Serve

- Sliced almonds

• Chopped parsley

Method

1. Turn up your oven to 450 degrees F (230 degrees C), and let it preheat for at least 15 minutes.

2. Dry the chicken by patting it with paper towels. Sprinkle paprika, salt, and pepper over it. Rub the spices well into the chicken.

3. Pour oil into a cast-iron skillet, and heat over a medium flame. Once the oil is heated, place chicken in the pan, and cook it until golden brown on both sides.

4. Throw in the bell peppers, onion, garlic, and tomatoes along with salt and pepper. Mix well. Turn off the flame.

5. Shift the skillet into the oven. Roast until the chicken is well-cooked inside.

6. Garnish with parsley and almonds and serve.

Quinoa and Black Bean-Stuffed Peppers

Ingredients

- ½ cup quinoa, rinsed

- ¾ cup water

- 2 large green peppers

- ½ can (from a 15 ounces can) black beans, rinsed and drained

- ¼ cup Monterey Jack cheese, shredded and divided

- ½ jar (from a 16 ounces jar) chunky salsa, divided

- ¼ cup low-fat ricotta cheese

Method

1. Turn up your oven to 400 degrees F (205 degrees C), and let it preheat for at least 20 minutes.

2. Pour water into a saucepan over high heat.

3. As it begins to boil, stir in quinoa, and lower the heat. Cover and cook until dry.

4. Cut a thin slice from the top of each pepper. Scoop out the seeds and any membranes.

5. Place the peppers in a microwave-safe baking dish with the cut side facing down.

6. Cook on high for 3–4 minutes or until the peppers are crisp and tender.

7. Set aside 3 tablespoons of salsa, and combine the rest of the salsa with cooked quinoa along with beans, 2 tablespoons Monterey Jack cheese, and ricotta cheese.

8. Fill this mixture into the peppers. Place the filled peppers in the baking dish, this time with the cut side facing up.

9. Top the peppers with the rest of the cheese.

10. Pop the baking dish into the oven, and bake for about 15 minutes or until well heated.

11. Serve with retained salsa (1 tablespoon per stuffed pepper).

Thai Green Curry with Spring Vegetables

Ingredients

- ½ cup brown basmati rice, rinsed

- ½ small white onion, diced

- 1 clove garlic, finely chopped

- 1 cup asparagus (cut into 2 inch pieces), chopped

- 1 tablespoon Thai green curry paste or to taste

- ¼ cup water

- 1 cup packed baby spinach, chopped

- ¾ teaspoon soy sauce or tamari

- 1 teaspoon coconut oil or olive oil

- ½ tablespoon fresh ginger, finely chopped

- Salt to taste

- ½ cup sliced carrots (¼ inch round slices)

- ½ can (from a 14 ounces can) coconut milk

- ¾ teaspoon coconut sugar or raw sugar or brown sugar

- ¾ teaspoon rice vinegar or fresh lime juice

- Red pepper flakes to taste

Garnish

- Chopped fresh cilantro

- Red pepper flakes to taste

Method

1. Place a pot of water over high flame. When it begins to boil, add rice, and cook until the desired doneness is achieved. Turn off the heat, and drain off the excess water from the pot.

2. Add the rice back into the pot. Cover with a lid, and set it aside for 10 minutes.

3. In the meantime, pour oil into a skillet, and heat over a medium flame.

4. When the oil is heated, add onion, garlic, and ginger and stir fry for a few minutes until onions turn translucent. Add a bit of salt while cooking.

5. Stir in carrots and asparagus. Let it cook for a couple of minutes.

6. Stir in curry paste, and continue cooking for a couple of minutes. Stir frequently.

7. Add coconut milk, water, and sugar and stir. Lower the flame and cook until vegetables are tender.

8. Add spinach and cook until spinach wilts. Turn off the heat.

9. Add vinegar, salt, soy sauce, and red pepper. Mix well.

10. Serve over rice. Sprinkle cilantro and red pepper flakes on top and serve.

Easy Brown Rice Risotto with Mushrooms and Fresh Oregano

Ingredients

- 1 ½ tablespoons olive oil, divided

- 1 clove garlic, peeled and minced

- ¾ cup brown Arborio or short-grain brown rice

- ½ cup parmesan cheese, freshly grated

- 1 ½ tablespoons unsalted butter, diced

- ½ teaspoon salt or to taste

- 2 sprigs fresh oregano, use only leaves, tear the leaves

- ½ small yellow onion, chopped

- 2 ½ cups vegetable broth, divided

- 6–7 ounces mushrooms, sliced and drained

- ¼ cup dry white wine (optional)

- 1 teaspoon tamari

- Freshly ground pepper to taste

Method

1. Place a rack in the center of the oven. Turn up your oven to 375 degrees F (190 degrees C), and let it preheat for at least 20 minutes.

2. Pour ½ tablespoon oil into a Dutch oven, and heat until the oil is hot.

3. Once the oil is heated, add onion and a bit of salt, and cook until light brown.

4. Add garlic and mix well. Cook until onions turn brown.

5. Pour broth and cover with the lid. Increase the heat to medium-high, and let the broth come to a boil.

6. Turn off the heat, and add rice. Cover the Dutch oven, and shift it into the oven. Bake for about an hour or until rice is cooked.

7. Start making the mushrooms during the last 15 minutes of baking. For this, add the remaining oil into the skillet. Place the skillet over a medium flame, and let it heat.

8. Add mushrooms and a bit of salt, and cook until mushrooms are brown and nearly dry.

9. Take out the Dutch oven from the oven, and add the rest of the broth into the pot.

10. Add butter, Parmesan, pepper, wine, salt, and tamari. Stir constantly for a couple of minutes or until the mixture has a creamy texture.

11. Add mushrooms, along with the cooked liquid. Add salt and pepper to taste.

12. Mix until the mushrooms are well distributed.

Harvest Rice Dish

Ingredients

- ¼ cup almonds, slivered
- ¼ cup uncooked brown rice
- 1 ½ tablespoons butter
- ½ tablespoon brown sugar
- 1/3 cup mushrooms, sliced
- Salt to taste
- 1 cup chicken broth
- ¼ cup uncooked wild rice
- 1 ½ onions, cut into ½ inch wedges
- ½ cup dried cranberries
- ¼ teaspoon orange zest, grated
- Pepper to taste

Method

1. Turn up your oven to 350 degrees F (175 degrees C), and let it preheat for 5 minutes.

2. Spread almonds on a baking sheet. Place the baking sheet in the oven, and toast for a few minutes as per your preference, about 5–8 minutes or longer. Leave to cool on your countertop.

3. In the meantime, add wild rice, brown rice, and broth into a saucepan, and heat over a medium flame.

4. When the mixture begins to boil, lower the heat and cook covered until dry.

5. While the rice is cooking, place a skillet over a medium-high flame. Add butter. Once butter melts, add onion and brown sugar, and cook until onions turn pink.

6. Lower the flame, and continue cooking until golden brown.

7. Add mushrooms and cranberries, and mix well. Cook covered until berries bulge up a bit.

8. Add orange zest and almonds and stir. Add rice, salt, and pepper and stir.

9. Serve hot.

Mexican Quinoa

Ingredients

- ½ cup fresh or frozen corn kernels

- 1 ½ cups cooked white quinoa

- ½ cup jarred salsa

- ½ can (from a 15 ounces can) black beans

- ½ tablespoon ground cumin

- A handful of fresh cilantro to garnish

Method

1. Add corn and black beans into a skillet, and heat over a medium flame.

2. Once the corn is tender, stir in cumin and quinoa. Heat thoroughly, stirring often.

3. Add salsa and mix well. Cook until dry, stirring occasionally. Turn off the heat. Let it rest for 10 minutes.

4. Stir lightly using a fork. Sprinkle cilantro on top and serve.

Ground Beef and Cabbage Rolls

Ingredients

- 24 cabbage leaves, whole

- 2 eggs, beaten

- 2 teaspoons Worcestershire sauce

- 2 cups cooked white rice

- 1/2 cup minced onion

- 1/2 cup milk

- 2 1/2 teaspoons salt or to taste

- 2 pounds extra-lean ground beef

- 2 cups canned tomato sauce

- 2 1/2 teaspoons ground black pepper or to taste

- 2 tablespoons lemon juice

- 2 tablespoons brown sugar

Method

1. Fill a large pot with water, and add a little salt to it. Heat over a high flame until the water is bubbling. Dunk the cabbage leaf into the boiling water, and let the leaf boil for at least 2 minutes before removing it from the water.

Place in a strainer, and pour some cold water over it to stop the cooking process. Allow to drain.

2. In a small mixing bowl, whisk together the eggs, milk, salt, and pepper.

3. In a large mixing bowl, combine the cooked white rice, chopped onion, and ground beef, and mix well. Pour the egg and milk mixture into the bowl, and mix well to prepare a filling.

4. Place about ¼ cup of this beef and rice mixture in the center of the cabbage roll, and tightly roll it up. Place these rolls into a slow cooker.

5. Combine the brown sugar, tomato sauce, Worcestershire sauce, and lemon juice together in a small mixing bowl. Pour this condiment mixture over the prepared cabbage rolls in the slow cooker.

6. Cover the slow cooker with a lid, and cook on the low setting for about 9 hours or on a high setting for about 4 to 5 hours.

7. Serve hot with a condiment of your choice.

Arianna Brooks

Ground Beef and Rice-Stuffed Peppers

Ingredients

- 2 pounds ground beef
- 1 cup uncooked long-grain white rice
- 1/2 teaspoon onion powder
- 2 cups water
- 12 green bell peppers
- 6 cups canned tomato sauce
- 2 tablespoons Worcestershire sauce
- 2 teaspoons Italian seasoning
- 1/2 teaspoon garlic powder
- Salt, to taste
- Pepper, to taste

Method

1. Turn up your oven to 350 degrees F (175 degrees C), and let it preheat for at least 20 minutes to 30 minutes.

2. Pour the water into a saucepan. Add the rice, and heat on a high flame until the water starts boiling. Reduce the flame, and place a lid on the saucepan. Let the rice cook for about 20 minutes.

3. Place the ground beef in a skillet, and heat over a medium-high flame. Cook the beef until it is well browned. Crumble the beef using a spoon.

4. Cut the tops of the bell peppers, and scoop the membrane and seeds from them. Place the peppers on a baking dish with the hollow side facing upwards. If needed, slice a little off the bottom of the bell peppers so that they can stand upright without tumbling.

5. Combine the browned beef, 3 cups canned tomato sauce, cooked rice, garlic powder, Worcestershire sauce, onion powder, pepper, and salt in a small mixing bowl. Mix well.

6. Spoon the beef and rice mixture into the hollowed-out peppers.

7. Combine the remaining 3 cups canned tomato sauce and Italian seasoning in a small mixing bowl. Pour this prepared sauce over the hollowed-out peppers stuffed with the beef and rice filling, leaving a little sauce for basting.

8. Pop the baking dish into the preheated oven, and bake at 350 degrees F (175 degrees C) for about an hour. Every 15 minutes, pop open the oven, and use a pastry brush to baste the peppers with the reserved sauce. Keep cooking until the bell peppers are tender to touch.

9. Serve hot!

Spiced Gluten-Free Cauliflower Pizza Crust

Ingredients

- 2 teaspoons chopped garlic

- 1/2 cup fresh parsley, chopped

- 2 eggs

- 1 cup Italian cheese blend, shredded

- 1 head cauliflower, coarsely chopped

- Salt, to taste

- Ground black pepper, to taste

Suggested Toppings

- Grilled chicken

- Bacon

- Sliced bell peppers

- Boiled corn kernels

- Sliced tomatoes

- Ground beef

- Sausages

- Grated cheese

Method

1. Turn up your oven to 450 degrees F (230 degrees C), and let it preheat for at least 20 minutes.

2. Place the coarsely chopped cauliflower in a food processor, and pulse on the grating blade for a few minutes until the cauliflower is well shredded.

3. Pour some water into a saucepan, and place a steamer on top of it. Heat the saucepan on high flame until the water is bubbling. Ensure that the bubbling water doesn't touch the bottom of the steamer.

4. Place the shredded cauliflower in the steamer, and cover with a lid. Steam the cauliflower for about 15 minutes or until the cauliflower is tender.

5. Put the cauliflower in a large bowl, and allow it to cool. Once the cauliflower is at room temperature, place the bowl in the refrigerator for about 15 minutes. Stir every 5 minutes.

6. Lightly spray the baking sheet with some cooking spray, and place a parchment sheet on the baking sheet. Spray the parchment sheet with some cooking spray.

7. Combine the parsley, garlic, Italian cheese blend, egg, pepper, and salt in a small mixing bowl. Pour this seasoning onto the refrigerated cauliflower, and mix well until all the ingredients are incorporated.

8. Pour the spiced cauliflower mixture into the prepared baking sheet, and spread the flour into the shape of a pizza crust.

9. Pop the pizza crust into the preheated oven, and bake for about 20 minutes or until the pizza crust is evenly browned.

10. Remove the crust from the oven, and cool before covering the crust with the condiments and toppings of your choice. Bake again for a few minutes to melt the cheese, and serve hot.

Delicious Garlic Butter-Topped Steak

Ingredients

- 2 pounds sirloin steaks

- 1/4 cup butter

- 1 teaspoon garlic powder

- 2 cloves garlic, minced

- Salt, to taste

- Pepper, to taste

Method

1. Turn up an outdoor grill to a high flame, and allow it to preheat for at least 20 to 30 minutes.

2. Place the butter in a small saucepan, and heat over a medium-low flame until the butter completely melts. Add the minced garlic and garlic powder to the butter, and mix well. Take off heat and keep aside.

3. Place a steak on a flat surface, and generously sprinkle salt and pepper on it. Flip it over and sprinkle salt and pepper on the other side, too.

4. Place the steaks on the preheated grill, and cook for about 5 minutes on each side for a medium steak. You may increase or decrease the cooking time, depending upon the doneness desired.

5. Once the steaks are cooked, transfer the steaks to warmed plates, and top with generous amounts of the prepared garlic butter. Let the garlic butter sit on the steaks for about 3 minutes.

6. Serve immediately with a side of boiled vegetables, mashed potatoes, or creamy corn.

Side Dish Recipes

A meal is only as good as its side dish, or so it is said. Like every superhero needs a sidekick, like every cheesy protagonist needing a funny wingman, every main dish needs a side dish to complement it! However, most side dishes contain a healthy serving of gluten, making it very difficult to find gluten-free versions. In this section, you will find some side dish recipes that are delicious, nutritious, and healthy!

Parmesan-Roasted Broccoli

Ingredients

- ½ head broccoli, cut into florets, discard the thicker part of the stems

- Salt to taste

- 2 tablespoons parmesan cheese, grated

- Pepper to taste

- ½ tablespoon olive oil

Method

1. Turn up your oven to 375 degrees F (190 degrees C), and let it preheat for at least 20 minutes.

2. Place broccoli in a baking dish. Sprinkle salt and pepper over it. Drizzle oil over the broccoli. Toss well, and spread it in a single layer.

3. Pop the baking dish into the oven, and roast the broccoli until light brown or roasted to the desired doneness.

4. Take out the baking dish from the oven. Sprinkle cheese on top.

5. Toss well and serve.

Greek Salad with Avocado

Ingredients

- 1 ½ tablespoons extra-virgin olive oil

- ½ teaspoon dried oregano

- Pepper to taste

- ¾ cup cucumber, cut into ¾ inch cubes

- ¼ cup red onion, thinly sliced

- 1/8 cup kalamata olives, sliced

- 1 tablespoon red-wine vinegar

- Salt to taste

- 1 medium tomato, diced into ¾ inch cubes

- ½ avocado, peeled, pitted, and diced

- ¼ cup feta cheese, diced

Method

1. Add oil, oregano, pepper, vinegar, and salt into a bowl, and whisk well.

2. Stir in the cucumber, tomatoes, onion, avocado, olives, and feta.

3. Cover and set aside for a few minutes for the flavors to meld.

4. Serve.

Cool Beans Salad

Ingredients

- ¼ cup olive oil

- 2 small cloves garlic, peeled and minced

- ½ teaspoon ground cumin

- Pepper to taste

- ½ can (from a 16 ounce can) kidney beans, drained and rinsed

- ¾ cup frozen corn, thawed

- ½ small sweet red pepper, chopped

- ½ tablespoon sugar

- ½ teaspoon salt, or to taste

- ½ teaspoon chili powder

- 1 ½ cups cooked basmati rice

- 2 green onions, sliced

- A handful fresh cilantro, chopped

Method

1. Add oil, garlic, cumin, pepper, sugar, salt, and chili powder into a bowl, and whisk well.

2. Add the beans, corn, red pepper, rice, green onion, and cilantro. Toss well.

3. Refrigerate until use.

Sautéed Mushrooms

Ingredients

- ½ tablespoon butter

- ¼ teaspoon seasoned salt

- ¾ cup sliced button mushrooms

Method

1. Add butter into a skillet and place over medium flame. When butter melts, stir in mushrooms and seasoned salt, and cook until mushrooms turn brown and tender.

2. Serve hot.

Roasted Onions

Ingredients

- 2 medium unpeeled yellow onions, halved

- Salt to taste

- 1 tablespoon olive oil

- Freshly ground pepper to taste

- Balsamic vinegar to taste

Method

1. Place the rack at the bottom position of the oven. Turn up your oven to 425 degrees F (220 degrees C), and let it preheat for at least 20 minutes.

2. Sprinkle salt and pepper over the onion halves, and place on a baking sheet with the cut side facing down. Be generous with the salt and pepper.

3. Pop the baking sheet in the oven, and roast for about 25–30 minutes or until browned as per your preference.

4. Trickle balsamic vinegar over the onions and serve.

Purple Beet, Carrot, and Onion Medley

Ingredients

- 1 ½ beets, sliced

- ½ cup red onions, sliced

- Coarse salt to taste

- 1 ½ large purple carrots, sliced

- 1 ½ tablespoons apple cider vinegar

- Pepper to taste

Method

1. Turn up your oven to 400 degrees F (205 degrees C), and let it preheat for at least 20 minutes.

2. Add the vegetables into a casserole dish. Drizzle vinegar over it, and toss well.

3. Sprinkle salt and pepper, and toss well. Keep the dish covered with aluminum foil.

4. Pop the casserole dish in the oven, and bake until vegetables are cooked.

Sautéed Spinach

Ingredients

- 8.8 ounces spinach

- ½ tablespoon olive oil

- 1 clove garlic, minced or grated

- Pine nuts, to garnish

- Herbs of your choice

- Spices of your choice

- 1 tablespoon butter (optional)

- Lemon juice to taste (optional)

Method

1. Pour oil into a skillet, and heat over a medium flame until hot.

2. Add garlic, and stir for a few seconds until aromatic.

3. Stir in the spinach, and cook covered until spinach wilts. Add herbs and spices of your choice. Mix well.

4. Add butter now if using and stir.

5. Garnish with pine nuts, and serve with a drizzle of lemon juice if desired.

Gluten-Free Creamy Corn

Ingredients

- 10 teaspoons butter

- ¾ cup cream cheese

- 1 1/4 teaspoons white sugar

- 1 cup corn kernels

- 10 teaspoons milk

- Salt, to taste

- Pepper, to taste

Method

1. Combine the butter and cream cheese in a small bowl. Slowly add in the milk, little by little, and blend using a whisk or an electronic blender until smooth.

2. Add the sugar to the butter, cream cheese, and milk mixture, and mix well until the sugar dissolves.

3. Pour this mixture into a slow cooker. Add the corn kernels, and lightly mix. Add in the salt and pepper. Taste and season accordingly.

4. Cover the slow cooker with the lid, and cook on low for about 6 hours or on high for about 4 hours.

5. Serve with a rack of roasted lamb or a portion of grilled chicken!

Buttery and Sweet Sautéed Apples

Ingredients

- 2 large tart apples

- 2 tablespoons butter

- 1/4 cup cold water

- 1 teaspoon cornstarch

- 1/4 teaspoon ground cinnamon

- 1/4 cup brown sugar

Method

1. Peel the apples, and remove the core. Cut the apples into slices about ¼ inches thick.

2. Place the butter in a large saucepan or skillet, and heat over a medium-high flame until the butter melts. Add the apple slices to the melted butter, and keep cooking until the apple slices are extremely tender.

3. In a small bowl, combine the cornstarch with water, and pour this cornstarch mix onto the apples. Stir well.

4. Add the ground cinnamon and brown sugar to the saucepan or skillet, and let the mix boil for about 2 minutes, stirring continuously.

5. Take the pan off heat, and let the mixture cool a bit before serving.

6. Serve warm!

Spicy Black Bean and Quinoa

Ingredients

- 1/4 cup chopped fresh cilantro
- 1/8 teaspoon cayenne pepper
- 1/2 teaspoon vegetable oil
- 1 1/2 cloves garlic, chopped
- 1/2 onion, chopped
- 3/4 cup vegetable broth
- 1/4 cup quinoa
- 1/2 teaspoon ground cumin
- Salt, to taste
- Ground black pepper, to taste
- 2 cups black beans, soaked overnight and drained
- 1/2 cup frozen corn kernels

Method

1. Pour the oil into a saucepan, and heat over a medium-high flame until the oil is heated. Add the onion and garlic to the hot oil, and cook until they have browned lightly after about 10 minutes.

2. Add the quinoa to this onion and garlic mixture, and pour the vegetable broth into the saucepan. Sprinkle the cayenne pepper, cumin, pepper, and salt onto the mix and taste. Adjust seasoning accordingly.

3. Heat over a high flame, and bring the mixture to a boil. Cover the saucepan with a lid, and lower the heat. Cook the quinoa for about 20 minutes or until it absorbs all the broth.

4. Add the frozen corn kernels to the saucepan, and continue cooking the broth until the frozen corn kernels thaw out and become tender. This should take about 5 minutes.

5. Add the soaked black beans and cilantro to the quinoa mixture, and mix well to combine.

6. Heat for a few more minutes, and serve hot!

Dessert Recipes

Desserts on a diet? No, you are not dreaming! Gluten-free desserts are just the cherry on the cake! Finding gluten-free desserts is like looking for a needle in a haystack – time-consuming, arduous, and very disappointing. So, here are a few recipes that will help you make a bunch of delicious gluten-free desserts that will have you licking your lips.

Gluten-Free Peach Cobbler

Ingredients

For Biscuits

- 1 cup gluten-free all-purpose flour

- 1/8 teaspoon baking soda

- 2 teaspoons baking powder

- 1 ½ teaspoons cold unsalted butter, cubed

- 1 small egg

- 1 teaspoon lemon juice

- 1 tablespoon sugar

- 1/8 teaspoon salt

- ¼ cup buttermilk

- 1 tablespoon canola oil

For Peach Filling

- 3 tablespoons sugar

- ½ teaspoon ground cinnamon

- 1/8 teaspoon salt

- ½ tablespoon lemon juice

- 1 tablespoon cornstarch

- ¼ teaspoon ground ginger

- 4 cups peeled sliced peaches (about 2 pounds)

Method

1. For biscuits: Turn up your oven to 425 degrees F (220 degrees C), and let it preheat for at least 20 minutes.

2. Prepare a baking sheet by lining it with aluminum foil. Prepare a small baking dish by spraying some cooking spray into the dish. Place the baking dish on the baking sheet.

3. To mix the dry ingredients, combine flour, baking soda, baking powder, sugar, and salt in a mixing bowl.

4. Add butter, and cut it into the mixture with a pastry cutter until coarse crumbs are formed. You can use a fork to cut the butter into the mixture.

5. Add egg, buttermilk, lemon juice, and oil into a bowl. Whisk well. Pour this mixture into the mixing bowl. Mix until well combined and the dough is formed. Keep the dough covered with cling wrap. Set aside for a good half hour.

6. For peach filling: Add sugar, cinnamon, salt, cornstarch, and ginger into a small bowl and stir.

7. Add peaches and lemon juice into another bowl, and toss well. Combine this with the sugar mixture. Transfer this mixture into the greased baking dish. Spread it evenly.

8. Pop the baking dish along with the baking sheet into the oven, and let it bake for about 12–15 minutes or until the mixture is bubbling.

9. Take out the baking sheet from the oven. Make 5 equal portions of the dough, and place the dough portions on the peach filling. Continue baking until the biscuits turn golden brown.

10. Once the biscuits turn golden brown, take out the baking sheet from the oven, and let it cool until warm.

11. Serve.

Caramel Delight Energy Balls

Ingredients

- 2 cups rolled oats

- ½ cup caramel sauce

- ¾ cup mini semi-sweet chocolate chips, divided

- 1 cup unsweetened, unsalted almond butter

- ½ teaspoon salt

- ¾ cup unsweetened shredded coconut, divided

Method

1. Add oats, caramel sauce, ½ the chocolate chips, almond butter, half the coconut, and salt into a bowl, and stir well.

2. Take out heaping tablespoonfuls of the mixture, and shape into balls.

3. Toast the remaining coconut in a pan until golden brown. Place the coconut on a plate.

4. Add remaining chocolate into a microwave-safe bowl. Cook in a microwave for about 30 seconds. Whisk until smooth. If the chocolate has not melted, cook for another 10–15 seconds or until it melts.

5. Transfer the chocolate into a piping bag. Pipe the chocolate over the balls. Dredge the balls in coconut and serve.

6. Store leftovers in an airtight container in the refrigerator. It can last for 8–10 days.

Strawberry-Mango Nice Cream

Ingredients

- 4 ounces frozen strawberries, sliced
- 6 ounces frozen mango chunks
- ½ tablespoon lime juice

Method

1. Add strawberries, mango, and lime juice into the food processor bowl, and blend until smooth and soft-serve consistency.

2. Scoop into bowls and serve.

Avocado Chocolate Pudding

Ingredients

- ¼ cup nondairy milk of your choice
- ½ teaspoon vanilla extract
- 3 tablespoons cocoa powder, unsweetened
- 2 – 3 tablespoons pure maple syrup or to taste
- 1 ripe medium avocado, peeled, pitted, and chopped
- A pinch salt

For Garnish

- Fresh raspberries
- Cacao nibs
- Mint sprigs

Method

1. Add milk, avocado, vanilla, cocoa, salt, and maple syrup into a blender, and blend until smooth.

2. Divide into 4 dessert bowls. Chill until use.

3. To serve: Scatter raspberries, mint sprigs, and cocoa nibs on top and serve.

Cashew Cream Stuffed Strawberries

Ingredients

- ½ cup raw cashews, soaked in a bowl of water overnight

- ½ tablespoon maple syrup

- ½ teaspoon ground cinnamon

- ½ quart strawberries, cored

- 1 ½ tablespoons water

- ¼ teaspoon vanilla extract

- A pinch of sea salt

Method

1. Try to use strawberries of similar size.

2. Blend together cashews, maple syrup, cinnamon, water, vanilla, and sea salt into a blender, and blend until smooth. Add a few more drops of water if the mixture is not blending well.

3. Transfer this mixture into a piping bag. Pipe the mixture into the cavities of the strawberries and serve.

Coconut Strawberry Mousse

Ingredients

- ¼ can chilled, full-fat coconut milk

- ½ teaspoon sugar or honey

- 2–3 strawberries

To Decorate

- Strawberry slices

- Cocoa powder

- Coconut whipped cream

Method

1. Blend strawberries in a blender until smooth.

2. Add coconut milk into a bowl, and whip using an electric hand mixer for a couple of minutes.

3. Add blended strawberries and sugar, and blend until well combined.

4. Pour into a serving glass. Chill for an hour.

5. Garnish with strawberry slices, cocoa, and coconut cream and serve.

Arianna Brooks

Creamy Rice Pudding

Ingredients

- 4 cups milk

- ½ cup uncooked, long-grain white rice

- 2 tablespoons milk

- 1 teaspoon vanilla extract

- ½ cup white sugar

- 2 small eggs, lightly beaten

- A pinch of salt

- A pinch of ground cinnamon or to taste

Method

1. Pour milk into a saucepan. Add sugar and rice and stir. Cook on a medium-low flame. Keep it covered while simmering. Cook until rice is cooked. Stir often. Turn off the heat, and let it sit for 10 minutes.

2. Add eggs, vanilla, milk, and salt into a bowl and whisk well. Pour into the rice and stir.

3. Place the pot over a low flame, and keep stirring for a couple of minutes.

4. Transfer into a serving dish. Keep the dish covered with cling wrap. Make a couple of holes on the wrap.

5. Let it cool completely. Discard the wrap. Sprinkle cinnamon on top.

6. Cover once again with a new wrap. Chill for 7–8 hours.

7. Serve.

Chocolate Meringue Style Gluten-Free Cookies

Ingredients

- 1 1/2 teaspoons unsweetened cocoa powder

- 1 1/2 egg whites

- 8 teaspoons semisweet chocolate chips

- 1/4 teaspoon vanilla extract

- 1/8 teaspoon cream of tartar

- 1/3 cup white sugar

Method

1. Turn up your oven to 300 degrees F (150 degrees C), and let the oven preheat for about 20 to 25 minutes.

2. Whisk the egg whites until they are frothy. Add the vanilla extract and cream of tartar to the eggs, and keep whisking until the egg whites form soft peaks.

3. Gradually pour the sugar into the egg white mix, constantly whisking, until the egg whites form stiff peaks. The mixture should look glossy.

4. Add in the unsweetened cocoa powder and the chocolate chips, and fold clockwise.

5. Spoon about a tablespoon of the mixture, and place on a cookie sheet that has been sprayed with some cooking spray. Spoon the rest of the batter on the greased cookie sheet at 1-inch intervals.

6. Pop the cookie sheet into the preheated oven, and bake at 300 degrees F (150 degrees C) for about 25 minutes to 30 minutes or until the cookies start to crack.

7. Remove the cookie sheet from the oven, and allow it to cool for a few minutes before removing the cookies from the cookie sheet. Place the cookies on a wire rack, and cool completely before serving.

Gluten-Free Nutty Energy Bars

Ingredients

- 1 cup sweetened condensed milk

- 3 ounces semisweet chocolate chips

- 1/2 cup butterscotch chips

- 1/4 cup sliced almonds

- 3 1/2 ounces sweetened flaked coconut

- 1/4 lb unsalted peanuts

Method

1. Turn up your oven to 350 degrees F (175 degrees C), and allow it to preheat for at least 20 minutes to 25 minutes. Spray an 8 x 8 cooking pan with some cooking spray, or grease generously with some oil.

2. Place about 2/3 of unsweetened flaked coconut on the greased baking pan, and spread it all out to create an even layer on the bottom of the pan.

3. Create a layer of butterscotch chips on the coconut flakes. Evenly spread the chocolate chips on the layer of butterscotch chips, and top the chocolate chip layer with a layer of unsalted peanuts.

4. Gently pour the sweetened condensed milk over the layer of peanuts, taking care that you do not disturb the layers of coconut flakes, butterscotch chips, chocolate chips, and peanuts.

5. Place the sliced almonds in an even layer on top of the condensed milk. Top the almond layer with the remaining sweetened coconut flakes

6. Pop the baking dish into the preheated oven, and bake at 350 degrees F (175 degrees C) for about 20 minutes or until the layers solidify.

7. Remove the baking dish from the oven, and let it cool completely.

8. Cut the "bars" into evenly shaped squares.

9. Store the excess bars in an airtight container. Their shelf life is about 2 days when left out, but if refrigerated, they can be stored up to 10 days quite easily!

Gluten-Free Flourless Zingy Orange Cake

Ingredients

- 1 whole orange, with peel
- 1/2 teaspoon candied orange peel (finely chopped)
- A pinch of saffron powder
- 3 eggs
- 1/2 cup finely ground almonds
- 1/4 teaspoon baking powder
- 1/2 cup white sugar

Method

1. Place the orange with peels in a large-sized saucepan. Pour in enough water to just cover the orange, and heat on a high flame until the water starts bubbling. Reduce the flame to medium high, and let the orange cook in the water for about 2 hours. Check every half an hour to ensure that you do not run out of water and end up burning the orange.

2. Drain the water from the orange, and let cool completely. Cut open the orange, and remove the seeds. Place the orange flesh (along with the peel) into a blender or food processor. Blitz until it forms a coarse pulp.

3. Turn up your oven to 375 degrees F (190 degrees C), and let the oven preheat for at least 20 minutes. Spray a 5-inch round cake pan with some cooking spray. Place a parchment paper in the cake pan, and lightly grease again with some cooking spray or oil.

4. Place the eggs and sugar together in a large mixing bowl, and whisk using an electronic blender. Keep whisking until the eggs get a thick and frothy consistency and become pale.

5. Add the baking powder to the saffron.

6. Pour the orange pulp into the mix, and mix gently.

7. Slowly add the almond meal with the candied oranges, and fold gently.

8. Pour this prepared batter into the greased and lined cake pan.

9. Pop into the preheated oven, and bake the cake at 375 degrees F (190 degrees C) for about an hour or until a toothpick inserted in the center of the cake comes out clean and crumb-free.

10. Remove the cake pan from the oven, and allow the cake to cool in the pan for about 10 minutes before placing it on a serving plate.

11. Allow to cool completely. Serve with a few dollops of whipped cream and some crushed candied orange peel.

Arianna Brooks

Bonus Chapter – 16-Day Sample Meal Plan

To really kickstart your new lifestyle, I've provided you with a sample 14-day gluten-free plan. This is carefully designed to provide plenty of healthy foods – you will need to prep for scratch on some of them, but I do give you the recipes and a few tips on forward planning.

Week One

Prepping at the start of the week can save you a whole heap of time later on (recipes at the end):

1. Prepare the Zucchini Noodles and Turkey Bolognese for lunches on days two, three, four and five.

2. Prepare the Baked Omelet Muffins for quick breakfasts on days two, four, five, and six and as snacks for other days.

3. Make a whole batch of the Citrus Vinaigrette for the week.

4. Prepare the Avocado Yogurt Dip for days one, two, three, and four.

* = recipe included

Day One

Breakfast – 231 calories

- 1 serving of steel-cut oatmeal*

- 1 cup of fresh raspberries

- 1 tsp of brown sugar

Morning Snack – 106 calories

- 1 baked omelet muffin*

Lunch – 325 calories

- 1 serving of creamy tomato soup*

- 1 cup of cucumber, sliced

- ½ a large avocado, diced

Toss the avocado and cucumber in 1 tsp red wine vinegar and 1 tsp olive oil; season with salt and pepper.

Afternoon Snack – 121 calories

- 1 cup of small broccoli florets

- ¼ cup of avocado yogurt dip*

Dinner – 416 calories

- 1 serving of Cajun Salmon and Remoulade with Greek yogurt*

- 1 serving of potato salad*

- 1 cup fresh green beans, steamed

Daily Nutrition Totals:

1199 calories

68 g protein

123 g carbohydrates

35 g fiber

54 g fat

32 mg niacin

8 mcg vitamin B12

341 mcg folate

1608 mg sodium

Day Two

Breakfast – 254 calories

- 1 serving of baked omelet muffin*

- ½ cup fresh blueberries

Morning Snack – 171 calories

- 1 cup fresh raspberries

- 2 tbsp dry-roast peanuts, unsalted

Lunch – 311 calories

- 1 serving of zucchini noodles and turkey Bolognese*

- 1 apple, medium

Afternoon snack – 70 calories

- 1 cup small broccoli florets

- ¼ cup of avocado yogurt dip

Dinner – 370 calories

- 1 serving of vegetarian Niçoise salad

Daily Nutrition Totals:

1176 calories

58 g protein

105 g carbohydrate

30 g fiber

63 g fat

22 mg niacin

2 mcg vitamin B12

329 mcg folate

1815 mg sodium

Day Three

Breakfast – 214 calories

- 1 serving of steel-cut oats*

- 1 cup of fresh raspberries

- 1 tsp. of brown sugar

Morning Snack – 101 calories

- 1 cup of fresh, chopped pear

Lunch – 311 calories

- 1 serving of Zucchini noodles with turkey Bolognese*

- 1 apple, medium

Afternoon Snack – 63 calories

- 2 tbsp of avocado-yogurt dip*

- 2 stalks celery

Dinner – 512 calories

- 1 serving of polenta bowl with fried eggs and roasted vegetables*

- 1 serving of wilted garlic spinach*

Daily Nutrition Totals:

1201 calories

52 g protein

164 g carbohydrate

36 g fiber

44 g fat

19 mg niacin

2 mcg vitamin B12

525 mcg folate

1700 mg sodium

Day Four

Breakfast – 254 calories

- 1 serving of baked omelet muffins*
- ½ cup fresh blueberries

Morning Snack – 364 calories

- 1 cup of fresh raspberries

Lunch – 311 calories

- 1 serving of zucchini noodles with turkey Bolognese*
- 1 apple, medium

Afternoon Snack – 121 calories

- 1 cup of small broccoli florets
- ¼ cup of avocado yogurt dip*

Dinner – 430 calories

- 1 serving of Philly cheesesteak stuffed peppers*
- 1 serving of sweet potato fries, oven-baked*

Daily Nutrition Totals:

1179 calories

73 g protein

112 g carbohydrate

30 g fiber

55 g fat

29 mg niacin

3 mcg vitamin B12

307 mcg folate

2025 mg sodium

Day Five

Breakfast – 254 calories

- 1 serving of baked omelet muffins*

- ½ cup fresh blueberries

Morning Snack – 209 calories

- 1 fresh pear

- 2 tbsp dry-roast peanuts, unsalted

Lunch – 311 calories

- 1 serving of zucchini noodles with turkey Bolognese*

- 1 apple, medium

Afternoon Snack – 64 calories

- 1 cup of fresh raspberries

Dinner – 352 calories

- 1 serving of eggplant parmesan*

- 2 cups fresh spinach

- 1 tbsp. of citrus vinaigrette*

- ¼ large avocado

Daily Nutritional Totals:

1189 calories

54 g protein

125 g carbohydrate

36 g fiber

59 g fat

24 mg niacin

2 mcg vitamin B12

392 mcg folate

1633 sodium

Day Six

Breakfast – 254 calories

- 1 serving of baked omelet muffins*

- ½ cup fresh blueberries

Morning Snack – 101 calories

- 1 fresh pear, medium

Lunch – 430 calories

- 1 serving of mason jar tuna and chickpea salad*

Afternoon Snack – 62 calories

- 1 cup of fresh blackberries

Dinner – 375 calories

- 1 serving of Thai pork and rice noodles with cucumber*

Daily Nutritional Totals:

1222 calories

70 g protein

125 g carbohydrate

28 g fiber

51 g fat

27 mg niacin

2 mcg vitamin B12

258 mcg folate

1481 mg sodium

Day Seven

Breakfast – 292 calories

- 1 serving of banana pancakes*

- 1 cup of fresh raspberries

- 2 tbsp of maple syrup

Morning Snack – 78 calories

- 1 boiled egg (prepare in advance if you want)

- Pinch of salt and pepper for seasoning

Lunch – 430 calories

- 1 serving of mason jar chickpea and tuna salad*

Afternoon Snack – 62 calories

- 1 cup of fresh blackberries

Dinner – 348 calories

- 1 serving of BBQ chicken tacos and red cabbage slaw*

- 1/3 cup black beans, low-sodium variety, rinsed

- Pinch of salt, pepper, and crushed red pepper

Daily Nutrition Totals:

1209 calories

74 g protein

143 g carbohydrate

32 g fiber

27 mg niacin

2 mcg vitamin B12

211 mcg folate

1637 mg sodium

Recipes Week 1

These are the Recipes for Week One:

Steel-Cut Oatmeal

One Serving = One Cup

Ingredients

- 1 cup of plant-based milk or water

- Pinch of salt

- ¼ cup of steel-cut oats – make sure they are gluten-free

- Low-fat or plant-based milk for serving – optional

- 1–2 tsp of brown sugar, cane sugar, or honey for serving – optional

- Pinch of cinnamon – optional

Instructions

1. Mix the milk/water and salt in a small pan, and bring up to a boil

2. Stir the oats in, and turn down the heat

3. Cook for about 20 to 30 minutes or until they reach the texture you want, occasionally stirring

4. Serve with desired toppings

Baked Omelet Muffins

One Serving = Two Baked Omelet Muffins

Ingredients

- 3 slices of bacon, roughly chopped

- 2 cups of broccoli florets, finely chopped

- 4 scallions, thinly sliced

- 8 eggs

- 1 cup of cheddar cheese, shredded

- ½ cup of low-fat or plant-based milk

- ½ tsp of salt

- ½ tsp of ground black pepper

Instructions

1. Preheat your oven to 325°F

2. Lightly oil a 12-cup muffin tin

3. Cook the bacon until crisp over medium heat and remove to drain on a paper towel – leave the fat in the pan

4. Cook the scallions and broccoli in the bacon fat, stirring for about five minutes or until soft

5. Remove the pan from heat and leave to cool for five minutes

6. Whisk together the eggs, milk, salt, pepper, and cheese

7. Stir the bacon and broccoli mixture in

8. Divide between the muffin cups and back for about 25 to 30 minutes or until firm

9. Leave to cool for five minutes before removing from the pan

Creamy Tomato Soup

One Serving = One Cup

Ingredients

- ¼ cup of chicken broth, low sodium

- ¾ cup of tomato puree, no added salt

- 1 tbsp of cream cheese, low-fat

Instructions

1. Whisk the ingredients together in a microwave mug or bowl

2. Microwave for about 2 minutes on high power or until hot and creamy

Avocado Yogurt Dip

One Serving = Two Tbsp

Ingredients

- 1 large avocado, peeled and stone removed

- ½ cup of plain, fat-free yogurt

- 1/3 packed cup of fresh cilantro

- 2 tbsp onion, chopped

- 1 tbsp fresh lime juice

- ¼ tsp kosher or Himalayan salt

- ¼ tsp fresh ground black pepper

- Hot sauce – optional, to taste

Instructions

1. Put all the ingredients into a blender

2. Blend until smooth, and add hot sauce if desired

* Can be made in advance and refrigerated for up to two days

Cajun Salmon and Remoulade with Greek Yogurt

One Serving = 4 oz Salmon, Two Tbsp Remoulade

Ingredients

- 4 salmon fillets (approximately 5 oz each, fresh or frozen and thawed) – pin bones and skin removed

- ¼ cup of plain Greek yogurt, fat-free

- 1 fine chopped shallot

- 2 tbsp fresh Italian parsley, finely chopped

- 2 tsp cider vinegar

- 1 tsp horseradish, gluten-free

- 1 tsp Dijon mustard

- ¼ tsp sweet paprika, plus another 1/8 tsp, divided

- 1/8 tsp garlic powder, plus another ¼ tsp, divided

- Pinch of salt, plus ¼ tsp, divided

- Pinch of black pepper, plus 1/8 tsp, divided

- 3 tsp olive oil

Instructions

370

1. Stand the fish on a counter for 15 minutes to bring to room temperature

2. Whisk together the yogurt, parsley, shallots, horseradish, vinegar, a pinch of salt, a pinch of pepper, mustard, 1/8 tsp of garlic powder, and ¼ tsp of paprika; cover and set aside in the refrigerator

3. Pat the fish dry on both sides using a paper towel, and brush 2 tsp of olive oil over it

4. Season with the rest of the garlic powder, salt, pepper, and paprika

5. Heat the rest of the oil over medium heat and, when hot, place the fish in, skin facing up. Cook the fish, pressing down using a spatula, for about five minutes or until the underside has turned golden brown

6. Carefully flip the fish and cook, skin-side down, for about two to three minutes – the fish should turn opaque and be just starting to flake

7. Serve straight away with the Remoulade

The Remoulade can be made ahead of time and refrigerated for up to two days.

Potato Salad

One Serving = Approx. ¾ of a Cup

Ingredients

- 2 ½ lb red or yellow potatoes, cleaned and cut into ½ to 1-inch cubes

- ¾ tsp salt, divided

- ½ cup mayonnaise

- ½ cup plain yogurt, low-fat

- ¼ cup onion, finely chopped

- 2 tbsp Dijon mustard

- ½ tsp fresh ground black pepper

- 2 boiled eggs, chopped

- 1 cup of celery, chopped

Instructions

1. Add one to two inches of water to a pan with a steamer basket attached, and bring to a boil

2. Add the diced potatoes, cover with a lid and cook for about 12 to 15 minutes, or until tender

3. Spread the potatoes on a lightly oiled baking sheet, and coat with ¼ tsp of salt; leave to cool for about 15 minutes

4. Whisk together the yogurt, mayonnaise, onion, the rest of the salt, mustard, and pepper

5. Stir the celery, potatoes, and eggs in, combining to coat everything in the sauce

6. Serve straight away or refrigerate until the salad is cold

Make ahead and refrigerate, covered, for up to one day.

Zucchini Noodles and Turkey Bolognese

One Serving = 2 Cups or One Container

Ingredients

- 3 cups of turkey Bolognese (see below for recipe)
- 8 cups of zucchini noodles, about 3 medium zucchinis
- ½ cup of parmesan cheese, grated

Bolognese Sauce

- 1 tbsp olive oil, preferably extra virgin
- 1 large chopped onion
- 4 cloves garlic, finely minced
- 1 tbsp Italian seasoning
- 1 lb lean ground turkey
- 8 oz chopped mushrooms
- ½ tsp salt
- 1 can crushed tomatoes, approx. 28 oz
- ½ cup of chopped basil or parsley

Instructions for Bolognese Sauce

1. Heat the oil over medium heat in a large skillet

2. Add the onion, and cook for about 5 minutes or until soft, stirring

3. Add the Italian seasoning and garlic and stir, cooking for about one minute until fragrant

4. Add the mushrooms, salt, and turkey and cook for about ten minutes – stir the turkey, crumbling it, and cook until the mushrooms are cooked through, and the meat is not pink

5. Turn the heat up, and add the tomatoes; occasionally stir, cooking for about five minutes or until the sauce has thickened

6. Add the herbs and stir in well

Instructions for Zucchini Noodles and Sauce

1. While the sauce is cooking, divide the noodles evenly between 4 single-serve microwave containers (with lids) – each should take about two cups of noodles

2. Add ¾ cup of the Bolognese sauce to each container

3. Sprinkle two tbsp of grated parmesan over the top and seal each container

4. To reheat, open the vents in the lids and microwave until the sauce is hot and the noodles tender, around two to three minutes on high power

These can be prepared in advance and refrigerated for up to four days. If you don't have single-serve microwave containers, store in foil or lidded containers, and transfer to a microwave dish to reheat.

Niçoise Salad – Vegetarian

One Serving = Four Cups

Ingredients:

- 3 cups mixed spring greens
- 2 tbsp lemon vinaigrette (recipe below)
- ¼ cup fresh or frozen green beans, steamed
- ¼ cup baby potatoes, cooked and diced
- ¼ cup halved grape tomatoes
- 1 large sliced boiled egg
- ½ oz Kalamata olives, pitted
- 2 tbsp or ½ oz of low-fat Feta cheese, crumbled

Lemon Vinaigrette Ingredients

- 2 tbsp lemon juice
- ½ tsp finely minced garlic
- ¼ tsp dried thyme
- 1/8 tsp salt
- 1/8 tsp ground pepper

- ¼ cup extra virgin olive oil

Vinaigrette Instructions

1. Whisk together the lemon juice, garlic, salt, pepper, and thyme

2. Slowly whisk the olive oil until completely blended

Salad Instructions

1. Put the salad greens in a bowl, and toss with 1 tbsp of the lemon vinaigrette

2. Turn out onto a plate

3. Toss the potatoes and beans gently with the remaining 2 tsp of vinaigrette, and place on top of the greens

4. Serve with egg, tomatoes, olives, and crumbled feta

Polenta Bowl with Fried Eggs and Roasted Vegetables

One Serving = ¾ Cup of Polenta, One Egg, and One Cup of Vegetables

Ingredients

- 6 shallots, cut in half lengthways

- 3 tbsp extra virgin olive oil

- 1 lb asparagus spears, trimmed and chopped into pieces, approx. 2 inches each

- 6 oz cremini mushrooms, cut in half lengthways

- 3 tbsp balsamic vinegar

- 1 tbsp fresh thyme, chopped

- ½ tsp salt

- ½ tsp ground black pepper

- 2 cups milk

- 2 cups chicken broth, no salt variety

- ¾ cup instant polenta

- ½ cup grated cheese

- 4 eggs

Instructions

1. Preheat your oven to 425°F, and line a large baking sheet with tin foil

2. Spread the shallots over the pan, and drizzle one tbsp oil over them; toss to coat thoroughly, and roast for about 12 minutes or until light brown

3. Add the mushrooms, asparagus, thyme, pepper, vinegar, ¼ tbsp salt, and one tbsp oil to the pan; stir and roast for eight minutes or until the vegetables are tender but not overcooked

4. Whisk the milk and stock together in a large pan over medium-high heat; bring to a boil, and whisk the polenta in – cook until thick, stirring often, about four or five minutes

5. Remove the pan from the heat, and stir the parmesan in

6. Heat the rest of the oil over medium-high heat, and add the eggs, one at a time, keeping them separate and cooking until the whites are cooked but the yolks are a little runny, around two to three minutes

7. Divide the polenta between four bowls and top off with the eggs and vegetables; sprinkle the remaining salt on the top

Wilted Garlic Spinach

One Serving = Recipe

Ingredients

- 1 tbsp olive oil

- 1 clove finely chopped garlic

- 1 lb washed, stemmed spinach or 1 lb washed Swiss chard, leaves torn and stems sliced

- Salt and pepper to season

Instructions

1. Heat the oil over medium high heat; cook the garlic for around 30 seconds, stirring until golden

2. Add the chard or spinach a bit at a time, and toss until wilted, around two to four minutes

3. Season with pepper and salt to serve

Philly Cheesesteak Stuffed Peppers

One Serving = ½ A Stuffed Pepper

Ingredients

- 2 bell peppers, cut in half lengthways and deseeded

- 1 tbsp olive oil

- 1 large onion, cut in half and sliced

- 8 oz thinly sliced mushrooms

- 12 oz top round steak, sliced thinly

- 1 tbsp Italian seasoning

- ½ tsp ground black pepper

- ¼ tsp salt

- 1 tbsp Worcestershire sauce

- 4 slices of cheese, Provolone works best

Instructions

1. Preheat your oven to 375°F

2. Spread the halves of the pepper over a lightly oiled baking sheet, and bake for about 30 minutes or until tender but still in shape

3. In the meantime, place the oil over medium heat, and cook the onion for four or five minutes, stirring until it just starts to go brown

4. Add the mushrooms, and cook for about five minutes or until they release their juices and start softening

5. Add the steak, salt, pepper, and Italian seasoning and cook, stirring until the steak is just cooked all the way through; it will take about three to five minutes

6. Remove the pan from the heat, and stir the Worcestershire sauce in

7. Preheat your broiler to a high heat

8. Divide the mixture between the pepper halves, and place a slice of cheese on top

9. Broil the peppers, five inches from the broiler heat, until the cheese has melted and started browning, about two to three minutes

Sweet Potato Fries, Oven-Baked

One Serving = Recipe

Ingredients

- 1 sweet potato, peeled and chopped in wedges

- 2 tsp canola oil

- ¼ tsp salt

- Small pinch of cayenne pepper

Instructions

1. Preheat your oven to 450°F

2. Put the potato wedges in a bowl, and toss in the salt, pepper, and oil

3. Spread out in a single layer over a baking sheet, and bake for about 20 minutes or until brown and tender, turning once

Eggplant Parmesan

One Serving = One Cup

Ingredients

- 2 eggplants, about 1 lb each, trimmed and cut into ½-inch thick slices, crosswise

- ¾ tsp of salt

- ½ tsp ground pepper

- 2 tbsp olive oil, preferably extra virgin

- 1 cup onion, chopped

- 2 cloves minced garlic

- 1 can (28 oz) crushed tomatoes, no added salt

- ¼ cup of very dry red wine

- 1 tsp dried oregano

- 1 tsp dried basil

- 1 ½ cups of part-skimmed mozzarella, shredded

- ½ cup of parmesan cheese, grated

- Fresh basil, thinly sliced, for garnishing

Arianna Brooks

Instructions

1. Preheat your oven to 400°F, and lightly oil two baking sheets

2. Spread the eggplant slices over the trays and sprinkle ¼ tsp of pepper and ¼ tsp of salt over them

3. Roast for about 20 minutes or until the eggplant is tender

4. In the meantime, place the oil over medium heat, and cook the onion until soft, about four minutes

5. Add the garlic, and cook for a further minute

6. Next, add the wine, tomatoes, oregano, basil, the rest of the pepper, and ¼ tsp of salt

7. Stir and bring to a simmer, then reduce the heat and cook for about 10 minutes or until thick, stirring occasionally

8. Spread one cup of the sauce over the base of a baking dish, about 9 x 13-inch, and arrange the slices of eggplant over the top; spread another cup of sauce over the slices, and sprinkle half of the parmesan and the mozzarella over the top

9. Repeat with the rest of the ingredients for one more layer

10. Bake for about 25 minutes or until the cheese starts to brown and the sauce starts to bubble

11. Leave for about 10 minutes, and sprinkle with fresh basil to serve

Citrus Vinaigrette

One Serving = Two Tbsp

Ingredients

- 1 tsp orange zest

- ½ shallot, cut in quarters

- ¼ cup fresh-squeezed orange juice

- 2 tbsp lemon juice

- 2 tsp Dijon mustard

- ½ tsp kosher or Himalayan salt

- ½ tsp ground pepper

- ¼ cup olive oil

- ¼ cup avocado or canola oil, organic

Instructions

1. Mix the zest, juices, shallot, salt, pepper, and mustard together in a blender, or add to a bowl and use an immersion blender

2. Add the oils, and blend to a smooth consistency

Arianna Brooks

Make ahead and store in the refrigerator for up to five days.

Mason Jar Tuna and Chickpea Salad

One Serving = Four Cups

Ingredients

- 3 cups kale, chopped into bite-sized chunks
- 2 tbsp honey-mustard vinaigrette (see below for recipe)
- 2.5 oz tuna in water
- ½ cup canned chickpeas, rinsed
- 1 whole carrot, cleaned, peeled, and shredded

Honey Mustard Vinaigrette Ingredients

- 1 clove minced garlic
- 1 tbsp white wine vinegar
- 1 ½ tsp fine or coarse Dijon mustard
- ½ tsp organic honey
- 1/8 tsp salt
- 1/3 cup canola or olive oil
- Fresh ground pepper

Instructions

Blend all the ingredients together, whisking the oil in last

Salad Instructions

1. Toss the kale in the dressing, and place in a quart mason jar

2. Top off with the chickpeas, tuna, and carrot, and screw on the lid

3. To serve, empty the salad into a bowl, and toss to combine it all together

Make ahead and refrigerate for up to two days.

Thai Pork and Rice Noodles with Cucumber

One Serving = Two Cups

Ingredients

- 4 tsp organic honey

- 1 tbsp fish sauce

- 1 tbsp chili-garlic sauce

- 2 tbsp olive oil

- 1 lb pork chops, thin, boneless, trimmed, and sliced into strips of ¼ inch

- 6 sliced scallions, with the green and white parts separated

- 1 ½ tbsp fresh garlic, minced

- 1 ½ tbsp fresh ginger, minced

- ¼ tsp fresh ground pepper

- 8 oz vermicelli rice noodles

- 1 small cucumber, sliced thinly

- 1 ½ cups fresh bean sprouts

- 1 cup carrots, either shredded or julienned

- ¼ cup fresh mint, chopped

- ¼ cup fresh cilantro, chopped, plus a little extra for garnish

- 2 tbsp fresh lime juice

- Lime wedges for serving

Instructions

1. Combine the fish sauce, honey, and chili-garlic sauce together in a bowl

2. Place the oil over medium heat, and add the pork strips, garlic, scallion white parts, pepper, and ginger; cook for about three minutes or until the pork is no longer pink, stirring occasionally

3. Add the honey/sauce mixture and stir, coating the pork, scrape the pan to bring up the brown bits, and turn the heat down to medium low; continue cooking for a further two minutes, or until the pork is cooked all the way through, then remove from the heat

4. Cook the rice noodles as per the package instructions; drain them, reserving a cup of the cooking water

5. Add the noodles to the pan with the pork, then add the bean sprouts, mint, carrot, cucumber, lime juice, cilantro, and scallion greens; toss to coat them in the sauce

6. Add the cooking water a bit at a time, stirring until you have a loose sauce

7. Divide between four serving bowls, and garnish with fresh cilantro and lime wedges

Banana Pancakes

One Serving = 4 Pancakes

Ingredients

- 1 medium to large banana

- 2 eggs

Instructions

1. Blend the banana and eggs together to a smooth puree

2. Oil a large pan lightly, and place over medium heat

3. Add four lots of batter to the pan, using 2 tbsp per pancake

4. Cook until the edges start to look dry and there are bubbles on the surface, around two to four minutes

5. Flip the pancakes, and cook for a further one to two minutes

6. Repeat with the rest of the batter

BBQ Chicken Tacos and Red Cabbage Slaw

One Serving = Two Tacos

Ingredients

- ½ cup plain Greek yogurt, nonfat variety
- 1 tbsp sugar
- 1 tbsp lemon juice
- 1 tbsp cider vinegar
- ¾ tsp kosher salt
- ¼ tsp ground black pepper
- A dash of hot sauce
- 2 cups red cabbage, shredded
- 2 cups cooked chicken breast, shredded
- ½ cup light organic BBQ sauce
- 8 corn tortillas
- Fresh chopped cilantro for garnishing

Instructions

1. Mix the yogurt, lemon juice, sugar, pepper, salt, and hot sauce together in a bowl

2. Toss the cabbage into the sauce until coated fully

3. Mix the chicken and BBQ sauce together in a microwave bowl, and heat on high for about one minute or until the chicken is hot through

4. Heat the tortillas as per package instructions

5. Add ¼ cup of chicken to each tortilla, and top off with 3 tbsp of cabbage slaw

6. Garnish with fresh cilantro

Week Two

Here's how to prep for week two of your plan:

1. Make enough chili-lime chicken bowls for lunches on days nine, ten, eleven, and twelve.

2. Mix up enough citrus vinaigrette to see you through the entire week.

Day Eight

Breakfast – 223 Calories

- 1 cup of plain Greek yogurt, non-fat variety

- ½ cup fresh blueberries

- 1 tbsp walnuts, chopped

Morning Snack – 62 calories

- 1 cup of fresh blackberries

Lunch – 339 calories

- 2 servings of tuna salad spread*

- 2 cups of fresh spinach

- 1 tbsp citrus vinaigrette

Afternoon Snack – 64 Calories

- 1 cup of fresh raspberries

Dinner – 500 Calories

- 1 serving of salmon and asparagus in a lemon and garlic butter sauce*

- ¾ cup quinoa*

- 2 cups of mixed greens

- 1 tbsp citrus vinaigrette

Daily Nutritional Totals:

1197 calories

83 g protein

100 g carbohydrate

34 g fiber

57 g fat

22 mg niacin

7 mcg vitamin B12

579 mcg folate

10 mg sodium

Day Nine

Breakfast – 223 Calories

- 1 cup of plain Greek yogurt, non-fat variety

- ½ cup fresh blueberries

- 1 tbsp walnuts, chopped

Morning Snack – 62 Calories

- 1 cup of fresh blackberries

Lunch – 413 Calories

- 1 serving of lime chili chicken bowl*

Afternoon Snack – 64 Calories

- 1 cup of fresh raspberries

Dinner – 462 Calories

- 1 serving of BBQ chicken stuffed potatoes*

- 1 cup of steamed spinach

Daily Nutritional Totals:

1223 calories

92 g protein

149 g carbohydrate

35 g fiber

35 g fat

31 mg niacin

2 mcg vitamin B12

1405 mg sodium

Day Ten

Breakfast - 368 Calories

- 1 serving of peanut butter overnight oats*

Morning Snack – 21 Calories

- ¾ red bell pepper, sliced or chopped

Lunch – 413 Calories

- 1 serving of lime chili chicken bowl*

Afternoon Snack – 30 Calories

- 1 plum

Dinner – 387 Calories

- 1 serving of spaghetti squash stuffed with artichokes and cheesy spinach*

- 2 cups of mixed greens

- 1 tbsp citrus vinaigrette*

- ¼ large avocado

Daily Nutritional Totals:

1219 calories

56 g protein

153 g carbohydrate

36 g fiber

49 g fat

18 mcg niacin

2 mcg vitamin B12

477 mcg folate

1450 mg sodium

Day Eleven

Breakfast – 223 Calories

- 1 cup of plain Greek yogurt, non-fat variety
- ½ cup fresh blueberries
- 1 tbsp walnuts, chopped

Morning Snack – 64 Calories

- 1 cup fresh raspberries

Lunch – 413 Calories

- 1 serving of lime chili chicken bowl*

Afternoon Snack – 77 Calories

- 2 stalks of celery
- 2 tsp peanut butter

Dinner – 434 Calories

- 1 Serving of taco stuffed zucchini*
- 2 tbsp sour cream

- ¼ cup of Pico de Gallo

Daily Nutritional Totals:

1210 calories

83 g protein

107 g carbohydrate

28 g fiber

56 g fat

22 mg niacin

4 mcg vitamin B12

304 mcg folate

1726 mg sodium

Day Twelve

Breakfast – 368 Calories

- 1 serving peanut butter overnight oats*

Morning Snack – 30 Calories

- 1 plum

Lunch – 413 Calories

- 1 serving of lime chili chicken bowl*

Afternoon Snack – 62 Calories

- 1 cup of blackberries

Dinner – 334 Calories

- 1 serving of chicken and spinach pasta with parmesan and lemon*

Daily Nutritional Totals:

1208 calories

73 g protein

156 g carbohydrate

31 g fiber

37 g fat

29 mg niacin

2 mcg vitamin B12

331 mcg folate

1307 mg sodium

Day Thirteen

Breakfast – 368 Calories

- 1 serving peanut butter overnight oats*

Morning Snack – 64 Calories

- 1 cup of fresh raspberries

Lunch – 323 Calories

- 1 serving of turkey cucumber sub*

Afternoon Snack – 62 Calories

- 1 cup of fresh blackberries

Dinner – 383 Calories

- 1 serving of Pork tenderloin and peach salsa*
- 2 cups of mixed greens
- 1 tbsp citrus vinaigrette*

Daily Nutritional Totals:

1199 calories

71 g protein

123 g carbohydrate

36 g fiber

53 g fat

31 mg niacin

3 mcg vitamin B12

329 mcg folate

1283 mg sodium

Day Fourteen

Breakfast – 336 Calories

- 1 serving of banana pancakes*
- 1 cup of fresh raspberries
- 2 tbsp maple syrup
- 2 tbsp walnuts, chopped

Morning Snack – 72 Calories

- 1 cup small broccoli florets
- 2 tbsp hummus

Lunch – 323 Calories

- 1 serving of turkey cucumber sub*

Afternoon Snack – 62 Calories

- 1 cup of fresh blackberries

Dinner – 422 Calories

- 1 serving of salmon tacos and pineapple salsa*

- I serving of broiled mango*

Daily Nutritional Totals:

1214 calories

71 g protein

136 g carbohydrate

30 g fiber

49 g fat

32 mg niacin

6 mcg vitamin B12

345 mcg folate

1326 mg sodium

Recipes Week 2

These are the Recipes for Week Two:

Tuna Salad Spread

One Serving = 1/3 Cup

Ingredients

- 1 large mashed avocado
- 2 tbsp plain Greek yogurt, non-fat variety
- 1 tbsp lemon juice
- 1 tbsp fresh parsley, chopped
- ¼ tsp garlic powder
- ¼ tsp paprika
- ¼ tsp kosher or Himalayan salt
- ¼ tsp ground pepper
- 5 oz Albacore tuna in water
- ¼ cup of diced celery or onion

Instructions

1. Mix the yogurt and mashed avocado together and stir

2. Add the parsley, lemon juice, garlic powder, pepper, salt, and paprika to the mixture, and stir well to combine

3. Lastly, drain the tuna, and add it to the mixture; add the celery or onion, and stir gently

Salmon and Asparagus in a Lemon and Garlic Butter Sauce

One Serving = One Salmon Portion and Five Asparagus Spears

Ingredients

- 1 lb wild salmon fillet, center-cut and sliced into four equal portions

- 1 lb fresh, trimmed asparagus

- ½ tsp kosher or Himalayan salt

- ½ tsp ground black pepper

- 3 tbsp organic butter (do NOT use margarine)

- 1 tbsp olive oil

- ½ tbsp fresh garlic, finely grated

- 1 tsp fresh lemon zest

- 1 tbsp freshly squeezed lemon juice

Instructions

1. Preheat your oven to 375°F, and lightly oil a large baking sheet

2. Layer the salmon to one side of the sheet and the asparagus on the other side

3. Sprinkle salt and pepper over both

4. Place the oil, butter, lemon juice, lemon zest, and garlic over medium heat until melted and combined

5. Drizzle the mixture over the asparagus and salmon, and bake for about 12 to 15 minutes or until the asparagus is tender and the salmon cooked through

Arianna Brooks

Quinoa

One Serving = ½ Cup

Ingredients

- 1 cup quinoa
- 2 cups broth or water

Instructions

1. Add the liquid and quinoa to a pan, and bring to a boil

2. Turn the heat down, cover the pan, and leave to simmer for about 15 to 20 minutes until the liquid is almost absorbed and the quinoa is tender. Fluff with a fork before serving

Make ahead, and refrigerate for up to four days. Will also keep in the freezer for up to three months.

Lime-Chili Chicken Bowl

One Serving = Two Cups

Ingredients

- 1 cup quinoa, cooked
- 1 cup brown rice, cooked
- 1 lb chili lime chicken (see recipe below)
- 1 cup jicama, julienned
- 1 cup thawed frozen corn
- 1 cup Pico de Gallo
- 1 diced avocado
- ½ cup fresh cilantro, chopped
- Lime wedges for garnish
- Hot sauce as desired

Lime Chili Chicken Ingredients

- ¾ cup of plain yogurt, low-fat variety
- 1 tbsp chili powder
- 1 tsp lime zest

- 1 ½ tsp fresh lime juice

- 2 cloves garlic, grated

- 2 tbsp olive oil

- ½ tsp kosher or Himalayan salt

- 1 tsp ground cumin

- 1 lb skinless, boneless chicken breast, chopped into 1-inch cubes

Instructions

1. Mix the oil, lime juice, lime zest, chili powder, cayenne, cumin, garlic, and salt

2. Coat the chicken in the sauce, and marinate for a minimum of two hours or overnight in the refrigerator

Lime Chili Chicken Bowl Instructions

1. Preheat your oven to 400°F, and line a baking sheet in tinned foil

2. Place the chicken on the sheet in one layer, and roast for about 15 to 18 minutes or until the chicken is cooked through

3. Mix the rice and quinoa, and divide between four single-serve lidded containers

4. Add the chicken, corn, jicama, Pico de Gallo, and avocado on top, sprinkle fresh cilantro on, and seal

5. Refrigerate for up to four days, and serve with lime wedges and a dash of hot sauce

BBQ Chicken Stuffed Potatoes

One Serving = 1 Stuffed Potato

Ingredients

- 4 medium potatoes, russets are best
- 2 cups cooked chicken breast, shredded
- ½ cup low-salt chicken broth
- 1 ½ tsp organic butter
- ½ tsp kosher or Himalayan salt
- ¼ tsp ground pepper
- ½ cup cheddar cheese, shredded
- ¼ cup sour cream
- ¼ cup BBQ sauce
- ¼ cup scallions, chopped

Instructions

1. Preheat your oven to 425°F

2. Pierce and cook the potatoes in the microwave for about 20 minutes on medium – turn a couple of times to cook evenly; if you prefer, you can bake the potatoes in the

oven for about 45 minutes or until tender and when cooked, turn out to cool a little

3. Place the broth and the chicken over medium heat until both are hot; put to one side and keep warm

4. Make a lengthways slit in each potato, pinching the ends so the flesh is exposed

5. Divide the butter among the potatoes and season with salt and pepper – scrape the butter in with a fork so it is incorporated

6. Top off with the chicken and cheese, and bake for three to four minutes or until the cheese has melted

7. Top with sour cream, scallions, and BBQ sauce to serve

Peanut Butter Overnight Oats

One Serving = 1 ½ Cups

Ingredients

- ½ cup soy milk or any other plant-based milk
- ½ cup old-fashioned rolled oats
- 1 tbsp maple syrup
- 1 tbsp chia seeds
- 1 tbsp powdered peanut butter
- Salt to taste
- ½ of a medium sliced banana OR ½ cup of berries

Instructions

1. Mix the milk, salt, syrup, oats, powdered peanut butter, and chia seeds together in a mason jar

2. Refrigerate overnight, and serve with berries or banana

Make sure that you only use gluten-free oats to be sure they haven't been cross-contaminated with barley and/or wheat.

Spaghetti Squash Stuffed with Artichokes and Cheesy Spinach

One Serving = 1 ¼ Cups

Ingredients

- 2 ½ to 3 lbs. spaghetti squash, sliced in half lengthways and deseeded

- 3 tbsp water

- 5 oz baby spinach

- 10 oz thawed frozen artichoke hearts, roughly chopped

- 4 oz cream cheese, low-fat, softened and cut into cubes

- ½ cup parmesan cheese

- ¼ tsp kosher or Himalayan salt

- ¼ tsp ground pepper

- Chopped fresh basil and crushed red pepper for garnishing

Instructions

1. Put the squash in a microwave dish, cut side down with 2 tbsp water

2. Microwave on high, uncovered, for about 10 to 15 minutes or until tender

3. Place the rest of the water and the spinach in a pan over medium heat until the spinach has wilted, about three to five minutes; drain the spinach, and transfer to a bowl

4. Preheat the broiler, with the rack in the top third of the oven

5. Scrap the squash out of the shells using a fork, into the bowl with the spinach, and place the shells on a baking sheet

6. Add the artichoke hearts, ¼ cup of parmesan, cream cheese, salt, and the pepper into the squash mixture, and stir it all in

7. Divide it between the two shells, and top ff with the rest of the parmesan

8. Broil for about three minutes or until the cheese has turned golden brown

9. Serve sprinkled with fresh basil and crushed red pepper

Taco-Stuffed Zucchini

One Serving = 1 Stuffed Half of Zucchini

Ingredients

- 2 large zucchinis

- 1 tbsp avocado oil

- ¾ lb lean ground beef

- 1 chopped medium tomato

- 1 bunch of scallions, sliced

- 1 tbsp chili powder

- 2 tsp ground cumin

- ¾ tsp salt

- ½ tsp garlic powder

- ¼ tsp ground pepper

- 8 tbsp Monterey jack cheese, shredded

- 1 chopped avocado

- 1 cup Romaine lettuce, shredded

- Pico de Gallo – optional

Instructions

1. Slice each of the zucchini in half lengthways, taking a small slice off the bottom of each one so they sit flat

2. Scoop the pulp out, so you have a ¼-inch shell, and chop up the pulp

3. Place the oil over medium-high heat, and cook the beef, scallions, tomato, chili powder, ½ a tsp salt, cumin, and garlic powder; stir to break the beef down and cook for about five to six minutes or until the beef is not pink, and then stir the chopped zucchini pulp in

4. Put the zucchini shells into a microwave dish, and sprinkle with the pepper and remaining salt; microwave, covered on high, for about two to three minutes or until tender-crisp.

5. Preheat the broiler to high, with the rack in the top third of the oven

6. Put the zucchini shells on a baking sheet, and divide the beef between them; sprinkle 2 tbsp cheese over each shell, and broil for about two minutes or until the cheese has melted

7. Serve with avocado, lettuce, and, if desired, Pico de Gallo

Chicken and Spinach Pasta with Parmesan and Lemon

One Serving = A Scant Two Cups

Ingredients

- 8 oz whole wheat or gluten-free penne pasta

- 2 tbsp olive oil

- 1 lb skinless, boneless chicken thighs or breast, trimmed if needed, and chopped into small bite-sized bits

- ½ tsp kosher or Himalayan salt

- ¼ tsp ground pepper

- 4 cloves garlic, minced

- ½ cup dry white wine

- Zest and juice from one lemon

- 10 cups fresh spinach, chopped

- 4 tbsp parmesan cheese

Instructions

1. Cook the pasta as per the package instructions; drain, and set to one side

2. While the pasta is cooking, place the oil over medium-high heat in a skillet with a high side

3. Add the chicken, pepper, and salt, and cook, stirring, for about five minutes or until the chicken is cooked through

4. Add the garlic and cook for another minute or until the garlic is fragrant; stir the zest, juice, and wine in, and bring to a simmer

5. Remove from the heat, and stir the spinach and pasta in; cover and leave to stand until the spinach wilts

6. Divide between four plates, and top off with 1 tbsp parmesan

Cucumber Turkey Sub

One Serving = 2 Sub Halves

Ingredients

- 1 large peeled cucumber
- 2 tsp brown or yellow deli mustard
- 2 tsp mayonnaise
- 2 oz sliced turkey breast, deli
- 1 slice Swiss or cheddar cheese
- 3 slices tomato
- 1 slice red or white onion
- Ground pepper for seasoning

Instructions

1. Slice the cucumber lengthwise in half, and deseed it

2. Lay the halves on a work surface, cut side facing up, and spread the mayonnaise and mustard over the top

3. Layer with cheese and turkey, and finish off with onion, tomato, and ground pepper

4. Put the two halves together, and cut in half to serve

Pork Tenderloin and Peach Salsa

One Serving = 3 oz Pork and ½ Cup Salsa

Ingredients

Peach Salsa

- 1 peach, cut in half and pitted

- 1 medium plum, cut in half and pitted

- 1 apricot, cut in half and pitted

- 1 slice onion, about an inch thick

- 1 tbsp olive oil

- ¼ tsp kosher salt

- ¼ tsp ground pepper

- 2 tbsp fresh cilantro

- 1 tbsp fresh lime juice

Pork Tenderloin

- 1 tbsp olive oil

- 2 cloves minced garlic

- ¾ tsp chili powder

- ½ tsp ground cumin

- ½ tsp salt

- ¾ tsp ground pepper

- 1 lb trimmed pork tenderloin

Instructions

1. Preheat your grill to medium heat, and brush all the fruit halves and the onion with the oil; sprinkle with ¼ tsp pepper and salt, and grill until grill-marked and tender, around three to four minutes on each side

2. Remove from the grill, and chop coarsely; transfer to a bowl, and stir the cilantro and juice in

3. Mix the garlic, oil, chili powder, salt, cumin, and pepper together and rub over the pork

4. Grill the pork, covered, turning it every 1 ½ minutes, until the internal temperature reads 145°F – it should take about 14 to 16 minutes

5. Transfer the pork to a clean board, and leave for 10 minutes

6. Slice it diagonally, and divide between four plates; top off with the salsa

The salsa can be made and refrigerated up to eight hours ahead of time

Salmon Tacos and Pineapple Salsa

One Serving = Two Tacos

Ingredients

- 1 salmon fillet, approx. 1 lb

- 1 tsp chili powder

- ¾ tsp salt

- 1 tbsp plus 1 tsp olive oil

- 5 cups of pre-packaged coleslaw mix

- ½ large lime, juiced

- 8 warmed corn tortillas (6-inch)

- ¾ cup of pineapple salsa (shop-bought)

- Chopped cilantro and hot sauce for serving

Instructions

1. Preheat the broiler to high heat with the grill rack in the top third of the oven

2. Place foil over a baking sheet, and lay the salmon on it, skin-side down

3. Broil until the salmon begins to brown and goes opaque on the sides – the thin part of the fish should be sizzling; it should take about five to eight minutes, and the baking sheet should be rotated once, front to back, to ensure even cooking

4. Sprinkle ¼ tsp salt and the chili powder over the salmon and drizzle 1 tsp oil over – brush it in, and continue cooking for another minute or two or until the spices are browning and the fish just begins to flake

5. Toss the coleslaw with the rest of the oil, the lime juice, and the rest of the salt

6. Remove the salmon skin and flake the fish; divide it between the tortillas, and top off with the salsa; serve with slaw, and garnish with hot sauce and cilantro

Warm the tortillas by stacking them and wrapping them in foil. Place them at the bottom of the oven while the broiler is on. Alternatively, you can microwave them for 30 seconds wrapped in damp paper towels.

Pineapple salsa can typically be found in the deli section of your grocery store. If not, you can purchase it in a jar, but choose one that has less than 80 mg of sodium in each serving and has no added sugars.

Broiled Mango

One Serving = Recipe

Ingredients

- 1 peeled and sliced mango
- Lime wedges

Instructions

1. Preheat the broiler, putting the rack in the top third of the oven

2. Place foil in a broiler pan, and arrange the slices of mango in one layer

3. Broil until it starts to brown, around 8 to 10 minutes, and squeeze the lime over the fruit before serving

Conclusion

If we were to make a list of things that the human digestive system is unable and not adapted to digest, gluten protein would probably be on top! This is an extremely sad fact, considering that wheat is one of the most omnipresent ingredients in our food today and is the root cause of a lot of health conditions. Most of these health conditions wouldn't have even existed if not for our extremely high consumption of wheat and products derived from wheat.

A lot of people have noticed a marked improvement in their health after adopting a gluten-free diet or even by just cutting wheat off their diet. So, if you are facing issues with your health, are suffering from celiac disease, or just aiming to lose some extra weight, all you need to do is cut the grains (and as a result, cut all the unhealthy foods) from your diet, and opt for healthier alternatives. Use the different options given in this book to help you do this. I assure you that you will see a positive change in your life almost immediately.

It is important to bear in mind that you cannot switch easily between diets. Thus, it can be difficult for you to ease into the Paleo diet or any gluten-free diet. Use the tips in the book to help you make this transition.

I would like to take this opportunity once again to thank you for purchasing this book, and I hope that you found the content helpful! Here is wishing you a happy and healthy life!

If you enjoyed this book, then I'd like to ask you for a favor: Would you be kind enough to leave a review for this book on

Arianna Brooks

Amazon? It'd be greatly appreciated! I want to reach as many people as I can with this book, and more reviews will help me accomplish that!

Thank you, and good luck!

FREE E-BOOKS SENT WEEKLY

Join <u>North Star Readers Book Club</u>
And Get Exclusive Access To The Latest Kindle Books in
Health, Fitness, Weight Loss and Much More...

TO GET YOU STARTED HERE IS YOUR FREE E-BOOK:

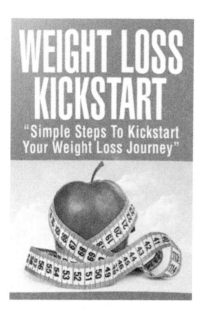

Visit to Sign Up Today!
www.northstarreaders.com/weight-loss-kick-start

Arianna Brooks

Resources

https://www.medicalnewstoday.com/articles/38085.php

https://www.verywell.com/five-different-types-of-gluten-allergy-562305

https://www.gluten.org/resources/diet-nutrition/the-gluten-free-nutrition-guide/

https://Paleoleap.com/exercise-and-Paleo-lifestyle/

https://www.glutenfreetherapeutics.com/living-gluten-free/medicine-research/social-side-living-celiac-disease/

https://www.healthline.com/nutrition/how-to-read-food-labels

https://www.fda.gov/food/new-nutrition-facts-label/how-understand-and-use-nutrition-facts-label

https://www.eatright.org/food/nutrition/nutrition-facts-and-food-labels/the-basics-of-the-nutrition-facts-label

https://www.pritikin.com/your-health/healthy-living/eating-right/food-labels.html

http://www.thepostgame.com/blog/training-table/201208/food-labels-harmful-ingredients-avoid

https://www.eatthis.com/healthy-food-substitutes/

https://pubmed.ncbi.nlm.nih.gov/15051613/

https://www.ncbi.nlm.nih.gov/pmc/articles/PMC3482575/

https://pubmed.ncbi.nlm.nih.gov/15554953/

https://pubmed.ncbi.nlm.nih.gov/22984893/

https://pubmed.ncbi.nlm.nih.gov/27211234/

https://pubmed.ncbi.nlm.nih.gov/18783640/

https://pubmed.ncbi.nlm.nih.gov/17990115/

https://www.ncbi.nlm.nih.gov/pmc/articles/PMC6266983/

https://pubmed.ncbi.nlm.nih.gov/24885375/

https://pubmed.ncbi.nlm.nih.gov/23126519/

https://pubmed.ncbi.nlm.nih.gov/24885375/

https://pubmed.ncbi.nlm.nih.gov/15051613/

https://pubmed.ncbi.nlm.nih.gov/24885375/

https://www.healthline.com/nutrition/signs-you-are-gluten-intolerant#TOC_TITLE_HDR_15

https://www.healthline.com/nutrition/gluten-free-diet#gluten-free-menu

https://paleoleap.com/exercise-and-paleo-lifestyle/

Printed in Great Britain
by Amazon